Clinical Approaches to Tachyarrhythmias

edited by

A. John Camm, MD

Volume 17

Clinical Approaches to Tachyarrhythmias (CATA)
Series Editor: A. John Camm, MD

Volume 1. **Mechanisms of Arrhythmias**
by Michiel J. Janse, MD

Volume 2. **Electrocardiographic Diagnosis of Tachycardias**
by Clifford J. Garratt, MA, MD, Michael J. Griffith, MA, MD

Volume 3. **Risk Assessment of VentricularTachyarrhythmias**
by Mark H. Anderson, MD

Volume 4. **Atrial Fibrillation for the Clinician**
by Francis D. Murgatroyd, MA, A. John Camm, MD

Volume 5. **ICD Therapy**
by Karl-Heinz Kuck, MD, Riccardo Cappato, MD, Jürgen Siebels, MD

Volume 6. **The Wolff-Parkinson-White Syndrome**
*by Carlos A. Morillo, MD, George J. Klein, MD, Raymond Yee, MD,
 Gerard M. Guiraudon, MD*

Volume 7. **The Long QT Syndrome**
by Peter J. Schwartz, MD

Volume 8. **Ventricular Tachyarrhythmias in the Normal Heart**
by John P. Bourke, MD, J. Colin Doig, MB

Volume 9. **Clinical Aspects of Implantable Cardioverter-
 Defibrillator Therapy**
by Martin Fromer, MD

Volume 10. **The Brugada Syndrome**
*by Charles Antzelevitch, PhD, Pedro Brugada, MD, PhD, Josep
 Brugada, MD, PhD, Ramon Brugada, MD, Koonlawee Nademanee,
 MD, Jeffrey Towbin, MD, PhD*

Volume 11. **Atrial Tachycardia**
by Michael D. Lesh, MD, Franz X. Roithinger, MD

Volume 12. **QT Dispersion**
by Marek Malik, PhD, MD, DSc

Volume 13. **Catheter Ablation of Ventricular Tachycardia in
 Patients with Structural Heart Disease**
*by Martin Borggrefe, MD, Thomas Wichter, MD, Günter Breithardt,
 MD*

Volume 14. **Atrial Flutter: From Mechanism to Treatment**
by Albert L. Waldo, MD

Volume 15. **Arrhythmias in Heart Failure**
*by William G. Stevenson, MD, Laurence M. Epstein, MD, William H.
 Maisel, MD, Michael O. Sweeney, MD, Lynne W. Stevenson, MD*

Volume 16. **Drug-Induced Long QT Syndrome**
by Yee Guan Yap, BMedSci, MBBS, MRCP and A. John Camm, MD

CLINICAL APPROACHES TO TACHYARRHYTHMIAS
edited by
A. John Camm, MD
St. George's Hospital Medical School
London, United Kingdom

Volume 17

Arrhythmogenic Right Ventricular Cardiomyopathy

by

Paul Touboul, MD
Professor of Cardiology
Chief, Cardiology Service
Director, Arrhythmia Unit
University Hospital Lyon
Lyon, France

Marjaneh Fatemi, MD
Attending Physician
Cardiology Service
University Hospital Brest
Brest, France

Futura Publishing Company, Inc.
Armonk, NY

Library of Congress Cataloging-in-Publication Data
Touboul, Paul.
  Arrhythmogenic right ventricular cardiomyopathy / Paul Touboul and
Marjaneh Fatemi.
    p. ; cm -- (Clinical approaches to tachyarrhythmias; v. 17)
  Includes bibliographical references and index.
  ISBN 0-87993-712-2 (alk. paper)
    1. Heart—Right ventricle—Diseases. 2. Myocardium—Diseases. 3.
Ventricular tachycardia. I. Fatemi, Marjaneh. II. Title. III. Series.
    [DNLM: 1. Myocardial Diseases. 2. Arrhythmia—complications. 3.
Ventricular Dysfunction, Right. WG 330 C6403 1993 v.17]
  RC685.M9 T68 2002
  616.1′24—dc21   2002070667

Published by
Futura Publishing Company
135 Bedford Road
Armonk, NY 10504

LC#: 2002070667
ISBN#: 0-87993-712-2

Every effort has been made to ensure that the information in this book is
as up to date and accurate as possible at the time of publication. However,
due to the constant developments in medicine, neither the author, nor the
editors, nor the publisher can accept any legal or any other responsibility
for any errors or omissions that may occur.

Foreword

When all is said and done, cardiac tachyarrhythmias account for considerable distress and untimely death. The arrhythmias may only be a consequence of a more serious underlying pathology, but irrespective of its pathophysiology an arrhythmia may pose a serious risk or a difficult medical problem. Tachyarrhythmias must, therefore, be diagnosed and treated with great care and expertise.

For too long the cardiologist and the arrhythmologist/ electrophysiologist have guarded their professional skills as secrets. In the past, the physician used the electrocardiogram and the electrophysiological study to establish accurate diagnoses, but the therapeutic consequences of these erudite diagnoses were negligible until the advent of electrophysiological surgery. Now the introduction of techniques of catheter ablation has catapulted cardiac electrophysiology into the medical headlines.

The mechanism of a cardiac arrhythmia is fundamentally important if therapy can be directed specifically toward that mechanism. Without knowledge of the target, the therapy cannot be aimed in the right direction. Some of our more successful therapies are "blunderbuss" treatments, such as amiodarone may well solve or suppress the problem. The cause of ventricular fibrillation is largely irrelevant to the corrective action taken by the implanted defibrillator. However, knowing, for example, that conduction through the right bundle branch is a critical component of bundle branch reentrant tachycardia identifies an easy target for ablation therapy. Similarly, knowledge about the cellular mechanisms responsible for the long QT syndrome suggests obvious and specific antiarrhythmic medical and surgical approaches to the treatment. This specific approach to therapy, suggested recently in the *Sicilian Gambit*, must sometimes be at arm's length—applying assumptions from tissue or animal models to the human clinical situation. On the other hand, the much more detailed deductions that can now be drawn from the surface electrocardiogram and from intracardiac electrophysiological recordings allow the electrophysiologist to make measurements and experiments directly on the culprit arrhythmia. The effect of therapeutic interventions may then be easily reassessed and further therapeutic measures can be instituted until all is well.

The aim of this series of monographs devoted to cardiac arrhythmology, made possible with the assistance of an educational grant from Medtronic, Inc., is to update the physician and cardiologist and all of those responsible for caring for patients with cardiac arrhythmias about the spectacular developments in diagnostic and interventional cardiac electrophysiology.

A. John Camm, MD, Series Editor
Professor of Clinical Cardiology
Head, Department of Cardiological Sciences
St. George's Hospital Medical School
London, United Kingdom

Editor's Preface

Twenty years ago, only a few astute physicians had recognized that a syndrome existed in which, unusually, the right ventricle became diseased and gave rise to ventricular tachycardia and sudden cardiac death. In severe cases, the right ventricle was dilated, sacculated, and very irritable. Ventricular arrhythmias ranged from ventricular premature beats to ventricular fibrillation, and the electrocardiogram showed classic features with right bundle branch delay or block and T wave inversion over the right ventricular leads (V_1 to V_3). A virtually pathognomonic feature was described: late potentials (epsilon waves), which were due to very delayed activation of sections of the right ventricle, were visible on the surface electrocardiogram and on recordings taken from the epicardial surface of the heart. This seemed to be a rare familial condition of little relevance. It was originally known as arrhythmogenic right ventricular dysplasia (ARVD), but it is now called arrhythmogenic right ventricular cardiomyopathy (ARVC).

Another much more prevalent condition was better known to cardiologists at that time: right ventricular outflow tract tachycardia (RVOT). Adolescents and young adults complained of sudden palpitations often provoked by exercise. The palpitations were seen to result from ventricular tachycardia with a typical QRS morphology resembling left bundle branch block (LBBB) with right axis deviation. No underlying heart disease was associated with the arrhythmia and its course appeared benign, although it was often sufficiently symptomatic (palpitations and some-

vii

times pre-syncope) to justify treatment with antiarrhythmic drugs, β-blockers, or non-dihydropyridine calcium antagonists. This more prevalent and apparently benign condition often masked patients who had ARVC.

The major differential diagnosis of a ventricular tachycardia with an LBBB-like morphology includes ARVC, RVOT, right ventricular cardiomyopathy, myocarditis, and myocardial infarction. Sensitive tools to spot early ARVC have only just emerged: fast cine computed tomography and magnetic resonance imaging. Both of these imaging techniques can identify fat deposition in the right ventricle (sometimes extending to the left ventricle in more severe cases)—the characteristic signature of ARVC. However, both techniques may also be of only limited value because of the frequent presence of high-density ambient ventricular premature contractions or salvos of ventricular tachycardia. Since ARVC is strongly familial in its occurrence, the examination of relatives may assist with diagnosis. The condition has a genetic basis, and one, perhaps two, genes for ARVC have been identified. As yet, however, routine genetic screening is not usually helpful to the clinician or the patient with putative ARVC.

Accurate diagnosis is important and the distinction between AVRC and RVOT is essential: RVOT is benign and it emanates from a single focus that can easily be ablated for symptom relief; ARVC may lead to sudden death, involves large parts of the ventricles, and generally requires treatment with an implantable cardioverter-defibrillator.

In this volume of the CATA series Dr. Touboul and Dr. Fatemi provide a comprehensive account of this syndrome that is now realized not to be "fine print," but relatively commonplace. Every cardiologist will probably encounter patients with this disease and this account of the condition is well worth the read.

A. John Camm, MD
Series Editor

Authors' Preface

Although first reported several decades ago, the combination of ventricular tachyarrhythmias and right ventricular diseases only triggered distinctive attention in recent years. In this view, Fontaine's pioneering work played a major role in defining a new clinicopathologic entity called "arrhythmogenic right ventricular dysplasia." Since that time, our understanding of the disease has known remarkable advances due to numerous studies devoted to diagnosis and therapy. Progress in knowledge has led us to revisit the concept of right ventricular dysplasia, which did not fit the complexity of the pathologic findings. Consequently, the various forms of the disease were included in the broader category of right ventricular cardiomyopathies. However, despite the data that have accumulated, the pathologic characteristics of the disease and the clinical expression as well remain debated. Similarly, the therapeutic options lack firm bases. Recently, the advent of genetics may have started a new era in the care of patients with arrhythmogenic right ventricular cardiomyopathy.

This book covers the whole spectrum of arrhythmogenic right ventricular cardiomyopathies. The reader will find the basic information about the anatomical substrate, the pathophysiologic mechanisms, and the clinical forms. A careful review of the diagnostic tests tackles the numerous available options ranging from the traditional electro-cardiogram to the most recent imaging techniques. Also discussed are the therapeutic tools, including drugs, and the nonpharmacologic approaches with special reference to the implantable cardioverter-defibrillator. As often as possible, the sections are accompanied by comments in order to help the reader draw the essentials and to guide him or her in daily practice. Besides rendering the book more attractive, the illustrations aim to clarify the text, which is of particular importance for the chapters related to pathology and imaging tools.

We believe that not only the specialist in arrhythmias but also any cardiologist will be well served by this book. No recent comprehensive publication has been devoted to this familiar but nevertheless ill-known disease. This work has given us the opportunity to gather and also to update the acquired knowledge in the field of arrhythmo-genic right ventricular cardiomyopathy. We hope it will meet the expectations of the reader.

Paul Touboul, MD
Marjaneh Fatemi, MD

Contents

Foreword... v
Editor's Preface.. vii
Authors' Preface ix

Introduction.. 1
Definition.. 2
Epidemiology.. 4
Pathology 5
   Macroscopic Aspect.. 5
   Histopathology.. 6
   Limits of Pathologic Diagnosis 11
   Pathogenesis.. 12
Clinical Presentation 14
   Ventricular Rhythm Disorders........................... 15
     Ventricular Ectopies/Tachycardia 16
     Sudden Death Due to Ventricular Fibrillation 22
   Other Arrhythmic Events 23
   Heart Failure 24
   Chest Pain 26
   Latent Forms 27
Diagnostic Tools 27
   Physical Examination 27
   Chest X-Ray.. 28
   ECG in Sinus Rhythm 28
   Exercise Stress Test 33

Signal-Averaged ECG... 35
Isoproterenol Testing.. 38
Electrophysiologic Study 39
Echocardiographic Findings 43
Endomyocardial Biopsy 46
Right Contrast Ventriculography 46
Radionuclide Angiography and Computed
  Tomography 47
^{123}I-Meta-Iodobenzylguanidine Scintigraphy........... 50
Magnetic Resonance Imaging.................................... 53
Genetics 53
Clinical Approach to ARVC 55
Differential Diagnosis.. 57
Right Ventricular Outflow Tract Tachycardia.......... 57
Uhl's Disease.. 59
Brugada Syndrome 59
Generalized Cardiomyopathy.................................... 60
Natural History and Prognosis 61
Therapy 64
Pharmacologic Therapy.. 65
Radiofrequency Catheter Ablation........................... 67
Surgical Disconnection of the Right Ventricle 68
Internal Cardioverter-Defibrillator 69
Treatment of ARVC Associated with Right or
  Biventricular Heart Failure 70
Prevention... 71
International Registry... 72
Conclusion.. 73

References.. 76
Index 89

Introduction

The myocardial diseases of the right ventricle have only emerged as autonomic clinical entities in the last few decades. Thus far, occasional pathologic reports had drawn attention to macroscopic abnormalities of the right ventricle, the most striking one consisting of extreme thinning of the wall resulting from deprivation of muscular fibers. In light of this, in 1905 Osler introduced the term "parchment heart" to describe this peculiar aspect of such hearts.[1] The clinical counterpart, however, remained ill known and no bridge existed between pathology and bedside. The first clinicopathologic documentation of right ventricular disease was presented by Uhl in 1952.[2] The case concerned a 8-month-old infant who had died of congestive heart failure. The main finding at pathologic examination was an "almost total absence of myocardium of the right ventricle." Thus, for the first time a correlation could be established between clinical course and right ventricular anomalies. The disease seemed to be restricted to infancy and responsible for early mortality. Several years later the concept of myocardial disease saw remarkable developments related to the discovery of new clinical forms occurring in adults and unveiled by cardiac arrhythmias. Reports of lethal arrhythmias attributed to Uhl's disease emerged.[3] Moreover, special attention was paid to patients suffering from drug-refractory, sustained ventricular arrhythmias in the context of an apparently normal heart. Fontaine et al.[4] were the first to stress the potential role of a right ventricular substrate in this subset of patients; their pioneering work is to be hailed. The initial report dealt with six patients who had developed recurrent ventricular tachycardia episodes and in whom complete investigation could identify dilatation and wall motion abnormalities of the right ventricle as the sole cause

1

of clinical manifestations. Three patients had antitachy-cardia surgery, which actually led to the recognition of the anatomical aspect of the disease, i.e., an unusual fatty appearance of the right ventricular free wall. The term "arrhythmogenic right ventricular dysplasia" (ARVD) was then proposed. This term took into account the potential for malignant rhythm disorders associated with the myocardial changes.[5] A new disease had emerged on the clinical stage, and years of intense research ensued to better characterize this entity. While diagnostic tools were refined, the most important contribution was provided by the pathologists whose findings were essential to identify subsets and to shed new insight into pathogenesis. In this view, the studies conducted by Thiene et al.[6] are milestones in the history of the right ventricular diseases. The concept of dysplasia was questioned, the anatomical data better fitting a myocardial process of the cardiomyopathy type.[7] More recently, genetics has entered the field of right ventricular cardiomyopathies, opening new and exciting ways for its understanding and management.[8]

Definition

Although still in use in the clinical setting, the classic denomination of "right ventricular dysplasia" should be replaced by "arrhythmogenic right ventricular cardiomyopathy" (ARVC), a term that suggests a myocardial involvement of the right ventricle in a broad sense without any reference to mechanism.[7] Two concepts are included: First, there is a myocardial process confined within the right ventricle. This right ventricular anomaly is an exclusive, or at least predominant, cause of clinical disorders. Moreover, ventricular arrhythmias are commonly present in relation to the myocardial substrate. This substrate is thus called arrhythmogenic because of its ability to generate rapid ventricular rhythms. Positively diagnosing ARVC consists of linking ventricular rhythm disorders to primary right ventricular alterations; however, the identification of a myocardial involvement may be arduous in case of very localized changes. In this situation ventricular arrhythmias appear to evolve in patients with apparently normal hearts. The clinical picture is that of idiopathic ventricular premature beats or ventricular tachycardia. This emphasizes the gap existing between the definition of ARVC and the diagnostic capabilities. Moreover, some forms of the disease may not be arrhythmogenic despite a clear-cut pattern of right ventricular cardiomyopathy. Assuming that the potential for arrhythmias is herein present but latent, these patients can be classified as having ARVC, just like those with clinical rhythm abnormalities. The current limitations of the diagnostic tools and the lack of pathologic findings make it likely that a significant number of right cardiomyopathy cases go unrecognized. Conversely, borderline cases may lead to false-positive diagnoses. As a rule, except for pathologic reports, the physician deals with probability diagnoses carrying variable margins of uncertainty. Coexisting damage to the left ventricle does not preclude the diagnosis of right ventricle cardiomyopathy if the right-sided abnormalities are suggestive, predominant, and further supported by relevant clinical markers. The incidence of this association is likely to increase in the late stages of the disease.[7] Finally, even the histopathologic criteria are a matter of debate. Replacement of the myocardium by fatty and fibrous tissue is characteristic, but the limit between normal and abnormal infiltration is unclear (see next section). Thus, if ARVC is currently viewed as a true entity, uncertainties still exist regarding the contours and, as a consequence, the recognition of the disease.

Epidemiology

The epidemiologic studies in ARVC are impaired by the lack of knowledge regarding the possible expressions of the disease. The notion of latent forms must be taken into account. This eventuality is supported by reports of ARVC-related sudden cardiac death in patients who were thus far asymptomatic.[6] The uncertainties of the diagnostic tests, as stressed in the following sections, still increases the difficulties of any epidemiologic assessment. Thus, incidence and prevalence of ARVC are currently unknown. The spectrum of the disease may range from latency to life-threatening events with in-between variable intermediate forms. Patients with a combination of symptoms, electrocardiographic abnormalities, ventricular arrhythmias, and evidence of pathologic changes of the right ventricular myocardium are likely to comprise a small subset. Since sudden death may reveal the disease, pathologic studies should be helpful to evaluate the role of ARVC as a cause of death. Such reports only provide indicative figures depending on the study frame, and their findings cannot be generalized. In this view, the results of a prospective Italian study of sudden death in the young[6] are of interest. This investigation was conducted in the Veneto region. Up to 20% of deaths in young people and athletes was attributed to previously undiagnosed right ventricular cardiomyopathy, which emphasizes the significant impact of the disease on juvenile mortality. In a more general context, ARVC was reportedly found in 5% of autopsies for unexpected sudden cardiac death.[9]

Moreover, ARVC may also be involved in cases of heart failure. The possible extension of the disease to the left heart is then misleading and erroneously suggests a dilated cardiomyopathy.[7] This illustrates the obstacles encountered by any attempt at quantifying the presence of ARVC in the general population. The fact that the entity is being underdiagnosed both pathologically and clinically is supported by the discrepancies between epidemiologic reports. The apparently high incidence of ARVC in northern Italy has not been mirrored in the United States.[10] A clustering of the pathologic process in some geographic areas is an alternative hypothesis whose determinants remain to be elucidated.

Pathology

Macroscopic Aspect

Knowledge of the pathologic aspects of ARVC has evolved greatly in recent years, after the initial findings of Fontaine et al.[4] were confirmed by more extensive studies by Thiene's group[6,7] in Padua. Gross examination may already detect the abnormal myocardial process (Fig. 1). The right ventricle may show thinning or, conversely, thickening of the wall. These aspects are either restricted to limited zones or, more often, widespread. Right ventricular enlargement remains mild and cases of marked dilatation are rare. Characteristically right ventricular aneurysms are often present. They are located at one or more sites: inferior, apical, or infundibular. Connected to each other, these locations draw what has been called the "triangle of dysplasia."[5] Macroscopic involvement of the left

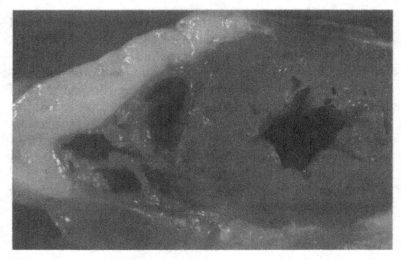

Figure 1. Cross-section of a heart with arrhythmogenic right ventricular cardiomyopathy. A massive, transmural fatty infiltration of the right ventricular free wall is apparent. Note the whitish aspect of the abnormal area as compared to the healthy myocardium.

ventricle is observed in about half of the cases with possible extension to the interventricular septum (Fig. 2).[7] Thus, the myocardial disease tends to strongly support the view that the exclusive right ventricular location is likely to be only part of a more global process. Moreover, valves, coronary arteries, and pericardium do not exhibit any abnormalities.

Histopathology

Histologic studies of these hearts reveal the pathognomonic changes underlying the macroscopic appearance. At the site of abnormalities there is a loss of cardiac muscle and its replacement by fat and fibrosis. The absence of myocardial fibers is associated with evidence of regional

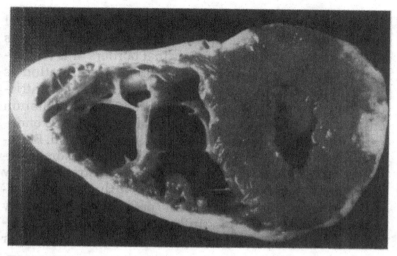

Figure 2. Cross-section of the heart from a patient with arrhythmogenic right ventricular cardiomyopathy who died suddenly. Note the massive and almost circumferential fatty infiltration of the right ventricle, with extension to the left ventricle.

or diffuse transmural fibrofatty infiltration. Surviving fibers can be observed inside the fatty tissue, and these strands are generally bordered by a thin rim of fibrosis.[5-7] Fatty degeneration of myocytes is likely the process that accounts for the histologic modifications. The lesions predominantly affect the right ventricular free wall and rarely the ventricular septum. Electron microscopy studies disclose no specific alterations in the myocytes. The amplitude of the fatty process and the respective part of the fibrous proliferation provide bases for defining two different histopathologic forms: a fibrofatty variety characterized by loss of myocardium with both fibrous and fatty tissue development, and a fatty variety in which myocardial cells are replaced almost exclusively by adipose tissue located intramyocardially and epicardially.[7]

In the fibrofatty form (Figs. 3 and 4), loss of myocardial cells is attributed to necrosis and apoptosis.[11] This results in fat formation and also fibrosis that borders or is embedded with cardiomyocytes. The fibrofatty infiltration is much more extensive on the epicardial side. Right ventricular wall atrophy associated with aneurysmal dilatation ensues. At this level, besides parietal thinning, the endocardium is thickened and the epicardium is whitish. Fibrofatty tissue development and myocardial fiber disorganization are likely to provide an appropriate substrate for slow conduction and reentrant ventricular arrhythmias. Myocarditis is a frequent finding in this pattern (Fig. 5) and may precede fibrosis.[10] Patchy inflammatory infiltrates composed of lymphocytes can be seen. It is unclear whether

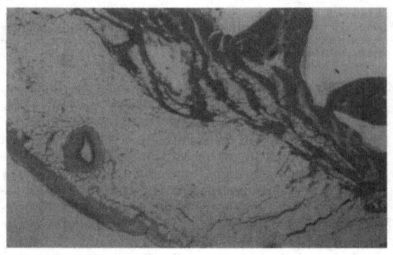

Figure 3. The fibrofatty form of arrhythmogenic right ventricular cardiomyopathy: the microscopic view of the right ventricle shows fatty infiltration of the epicardium adjacent to subendocardial fibrosis associated with myocyte loss. There are also areas of epicardial fibrosis. Magnification: 1×. Stain: hematoxylin-eosin-safranin. A color version of this image can be found on the color insert.

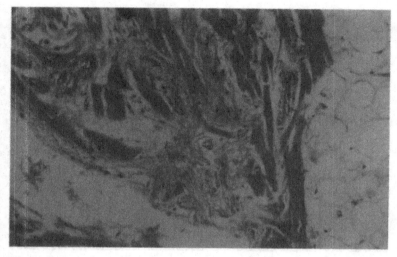

Figure 4. The fibrofatty form of arrhythmogenic right ventricular cardiomyopathy: adipose infiltration adjacent to islands of residual myocytes interspersed with interstitial fibrosis. Magnification: 10×. Stain: hematoxylin-eosin-safranin. A color version of this image can be found on the color insert.

myocarditis can be the primary cause of the fibrofatty degeneration, plays a role in the aggravation of the disease, or is a consequence of the spontaneous cell death.

The fatty variety (Fig. 6) is characterized by transmural fatty replacement of the right ventricular free wall frequently reaching the endocardium in the absence of fibrous tissue.[7] There is little inflammation, and absence of ventricular wall thinning. On the contrary, myocardial thickness is normal or even increased. Therefore, the incidence of aneurysms is low. Whether this form of ARVC carries increased risk of sudden death remains a conflicting issue. However, compared to the fibrofatty variety, no difference was noted in some reports regarding the occurrence of ventricular arrhythmias and mode of death.[10]

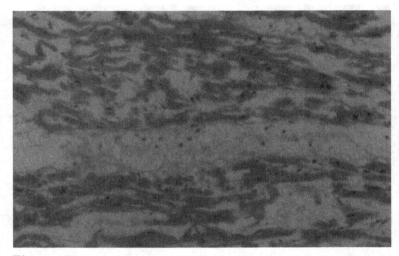

Figure 5. Arrhythmogenic right ventricular cardiomyopathy extended to the left ventricle: myocytolysis associated with interstitial
edema and lymphocytic infiltrates. Magnification: 10×. Stain: hematoxylin-eosin-safranin. A color version of this image can be found on
the color insert.

Involvement of the left ventricle and interventricular
septum appears to be exclusive to the fibrofatty variety.[12]
This notion further supports the idea that both pathologic
types of ARVC have different determinants and course.
Within the fibrofatty form, the cases with left ventricular
involvement may specifically exhibit lesions of the interventricular septum. Mural thrombosis is only observed
in this subset.[7] A higher occurrence of right ventricular
aneurysms has also been stressed. In biventricular disease,
the clinical course reportedly carries some characteristics
that are distinct from those of pure ARVC. More severe
damage extended to the left ventricle accounts for an increased rate of congestive heart failure.[7] Sudden death in
this setting would be less frequent, a finding which requires confirmation.

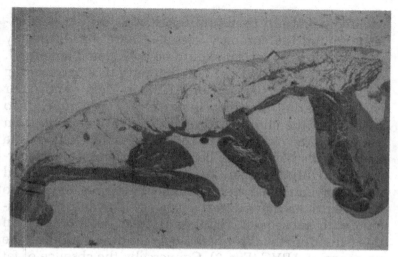

Figure 6. The fatty form of arrhythmogenic right ventricular cardiomyopathy: panoramic histologic view of the right ventricular free wall showing transmural fatty replacement. Note the epicardial coronary vessels embedded in the adipose infiltration. Stain: hematoxylin-eosin-safranin.

Limits of Pathologic Diagnosis

Pathologic features associated with ARVC can occasionally be misleading. Localized myocardial changes may elude gross examination. Whenever sudden death unexpectedly affects young adults, careful attention is to be paid to the right ventricle. Ultimately, the final diagnosis results from systematic histopathologic studies. Moreover, the notion of fatty infiltration is a matter of debate. It is well known that fatty infiltration of the right ventricle occurs in more than 50% of normal hearts, especially in the anteroapical region, in the elderly.[13] Fatty deposits are located predominantly in the subepicardium, or only infiltrate the outer third of the myocardium. The left ventricle contains fatty tissue only on the epicardium, particularly around the coronary vessels. There is controversy regarding how much fat should be considered abnormal. Angelini et al.[14] have claimed that fatty tissue exceeding 3.21% is highly suspect for ARVC in right ventricular endomyocardial biopsies. Burke et al.[10] reported up to 15% fat in the anterior apex of the right ventricle from normal hearts. According to Loire and Tabib,[15] fatty tissue that extends beyond the coronary vessels in the epicardium is highly abnormal. An additional problem is related to the biventricular involvement. Extensive damage to both ventricles may suggest a primary left ventricular disease with subsequent right ventricular deterioration. In this situation the histopathologic findings support the presence of ARVC (Fig. 2). Conversely, the absence of fat and fibrosis inside the left ventricular myocardium seems to exclude the diagnosis of extensive ARVC.[13] Due to these uncertainties, it is likely that the disease is largely misdiagnosed by routine autopsy.

Pathogenesis

The mechanisms underlying these morphologic changes are still debated. An analogy with Uhl's disease was originally postulated. The absence of myocardium was considered to be the consequence of a congenital structural defect of the right ventricular wall. Hence, the term "dysplasia" was proposed, implying maldevelopment as a cause of the pathologic abnormality. This term was used exclusively for years, and contributed to the recognition of the new entity.[16] However, unlike Uhl's anomaly, in which the ventricular wall is paper thin, in ARVC the distance between the epicardium and the endocardium can be normal or slightly decreased. Furthermore, given the progressive nature of the disease and the presence of foci of inflammation, degeneration, and necrosis, the term "cardiomyopathy" was subsequently preferred over "dysplasia."[17]

As knowledge accumulated with the emergence of new pathologic findings, it became obvious that the etiology and pathogenesis of ARVC required alternative hypotheses that better fit the myocardial changes. These hypotheses should account for the loss of myocardium and the substitution of fat and fibrous tissue. Two theories have been proposed. In the degenerative theory, the loss of myocardium is considered to result from progressive myocyte death related to some metabolic or ultrastructural defect of genetic cause. This theory is in accordance with the familial occurrence of the disease.[18-21] Interestingly, similarities exist between the pathologic substrate of ARVC and the skeletal muscular dystrophy observed in Duchenne's and Becker's diseases.[7] ARVC patients, however, do not seem to be affected by skeletal muscular abnormalities.

The other theory involves the role of inflammation. The starting point would be myocarditis. As a consequence of the inflammatory injury, disappearance of right ventricular myocardium would ensue associated with fat and fibrous tissue formation. The pathologic substrate of ARVC can then be viewed as resulting from a healing process following myocarditis.[22-24] The common occurrence of lymphocytic infiltrates supports the role of focal myocarditis (Fig. 5). However, the inflammatory cells are encountered almost exclusively in the fibrofatty variety and rarely in the pure adipose form. This further emphasizes the likely heterogeneity of the disease. Occurrence of infectious (viral) and/or immune myocardial reaction is invoked in the pathogenesis of the disease. In this view, it is noteworthy that the Coxsackie virus genome has been found in the myocardium of some patients with ARVC.[25,26] This is not in contrast with a familial occurrence, because genetic predisposition to viral infection eliciting immune reaction cannot be excluded. Similarly, genetic factors may also play a role in the site of cardiac involvement and account for exclusive right ventricular damage.

Clinical Presentation

The clinical spectrum of ARVC is remarkably wide ranging from paucisymptomatic forms to life-threatening conditions. The disease can even be latent, such cases being notably seen in families of patients with overt ARVC. Moreover, the clinical manifestations are often misleading. As previously stated, this accounts for major obstacles in any epidemiologic assessment, and more widely in the knowledge of the disease. In the clinical setting the diagnosis is rarely certain and carries varying degrees of probability. Many features have no specificity. The frequent occurrence of the disorders in teenagers or young adults leads to an underestimation of their significance. As a rule, ventricular arrhythmia is the index event that reveals the disease; however, the modes of expression are disparate. ARVC may mimic benign conditions in cases of isolated ventricular ectopic activity. Conversely, patients with sustained ventricular tachyarrhythmias are at risk of death. It should be remembered that the disease has been positively identified in patients presenting with drug-refractory episodes of sustained monomorphic ventricular tachycardia. Subsequently, ARVC was recognized as a possible cause of unexpected sudden death.[6] Thus

the arrhythmic events are prominent and truly characterize this cardiomyopathy. The hemodynamic deterioration
is rare and the cases with cardiac decompensation constitute a very limited subset.

Ventricular Rhythm Disorders

Ventricular tachyarrhythmias associated with ARVC
are the expression of the marked electrical instability that
characterizes the disease. The electrical disorders are related to the pathologic changes whose patterns favor the
fractionation of the ventricular depolarization wave.
Within areas of the right ventricle, the arrangement of the
myocardial fibers is disorganized by the fibrofatty infiltration. The ensuing irregular disruption of the myocardium
forms an arrhythmogenic substrate associated with inho-
mogeneous propagation of the excitation process. Localized unidirectional block may occur preceding the initiation of reentrant rhythms. This is supported by clinical
electrophysiology findings and occasional successful at-
tempts at suppressing ventricular arrhythmias by simple
surgical ventriculotomy.[4]

ARVC-related arrhythmias exhibit a propensity for
occurring during particular circumstances such as emotion or primarily exercise. These initiating conditions are
combined with an increased sympathetic tone. The role
of physical exertion is likely to imply both hemodynamic
and neurohumoral factors.[27] Increase of right ventricular
afterload and cavity enlargement may trigger ventricular
arrhythmias by stretching the right ventricular myocytes.[28] Progression of the disease from epicardium to
endocardium may also cause functional and/or structural
sympathetic denervation, decreased catecholamine reup-

take, and enhanced sensitivity to catecholamines accounting for arrhythmogenicity during sympathetic stimulation.[29]

Heart failure[30] can also be an aggravating factor. Increase of the filling pressures, ventricular dilatation, extensive fibrofatty infiltration, and activation of the neurohumoral system favor the emergence of abnormal rhythms. In this setting ventricular arrhythmias further deteriorate the clinical course and their management can be arduous because of the severe myocardial involvement.

Ventricular Ectopies/Tachycardia

Any pattern of ventricular rapid rhythm can be seen in association with ARVC, including isolated or paired premature beats, nonsustained tachycardia, and sustained tachycardia. Ventricular arrhythmias associated with ARVC are usually of left bundle branch block morphology,[5,6] indicating the right ventricular origin (Figs. 7 and 8). The QRS axis is inferior or normal when the ectopic beats originate from the right ventricular outflow tract, and superior when they arise from the apex or the diaphragmatic wall of the right ventricle.[31] Due to the frequent context of an apparently normal heart, the disorders may be misdiagnosed as "benign idiopathic ventricular arrhythmias."[31] Palpitations may draw attention to the premature beats. However, the clinical expression of extrasystoles in this setting is ill known and latent forms are likely to occur. ARVC-related ventricular premature beats are frequent, often paired or alternating with nonsustained tachycardia, and are present throughout the 24-hour day, with phases of exacerbation during daily activity. Patients presenting with attacks of ventricular tachy-

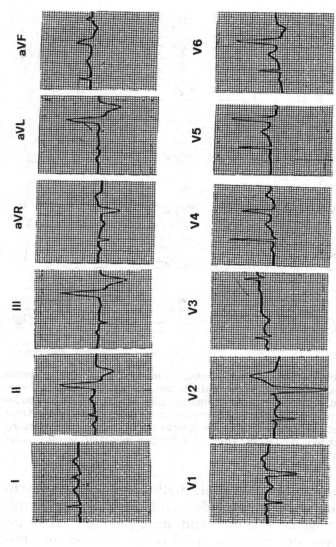

Figure 7. Twelve-lead electrocardiogram from a patient with arrhythmogenic right ventricular cardiomyopathy and recurrent episodes of sustained ventricular tachycardia. During sinus rhythm, numerous ventricular premature beats are recorded that exhibit a left bundle branch block pattern with a normal frontal axis. Note the inverted T waves in leads V_1 to V_3.

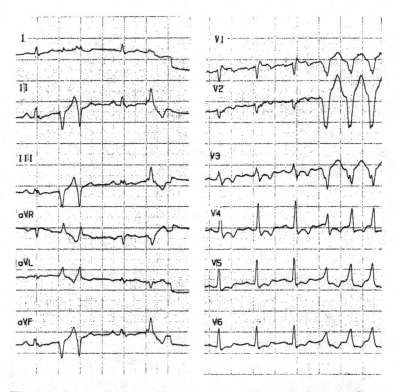

Figure 8. Twelve-lead electrocardiogram from a patient suffering from repeat ventricular tachycardia attacks in relation to arrhythmogenic right ventricular cardiomyopathy. Sinus rhythm is disturbed by frequent, polymorphic ventricular premature beats, with couplets and runs. Most premature beats have a left bundle branch block pattern with a left axis deviation. There is a T wave inversion in all precordial leads

cardia usually show in sinus rhythm numerous ventricular ectopies that provide evidence for an active arrhythmogenic substrate and are a potential target for antiarrhythmic drug therapy. This may support the presence of ARVC, since residual ventricular ectopic activity

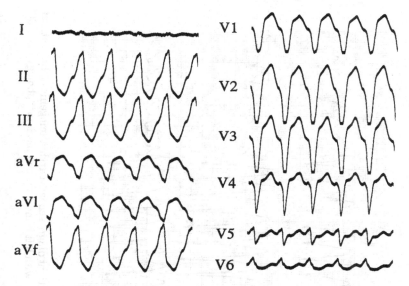

Figure 9. Twelve-lead electrocardiogram during ventricular tachycardia from a patient with arrhythmogenic right ventricular cardiomyopathy. Characteristically, the QRS complexes show a left bundle branch block pattern. Frontal axis is normal. Heart rate is 165 beats per minute.

is often lacking in patients with true idiopathic ventricular tachycardia.

Sustained ventricular tachycardia is a classic feature of ARVC. The tachycardia rate ranges from 150 to 260 beats per minute. As a rule, the wide QRS complexes are monomorphic with a left bundle branch block pattern and varied frontal axes (Figs. 9, 10, and 11).[5] However, rapid polymorphic ventricular rhythms can be observed that are viewed as heralding fatal events. Initiation of episodes of sustained ventricular tachycardias usually coincides with augmented sympathetic tone as demonstrated by the increased heart rate and the shortening of the coupling

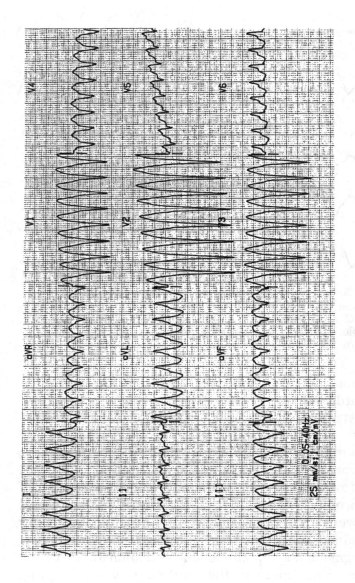

Figure 10. Twelve-lead electrocardiogram from a patient diagnosed with arrhythmogenic right ventricular cardiomyopathy. Sustained ventricular tachycardia with left bundle branch block morphology and −30° frontal axis. Rate is 250 beats per minute.

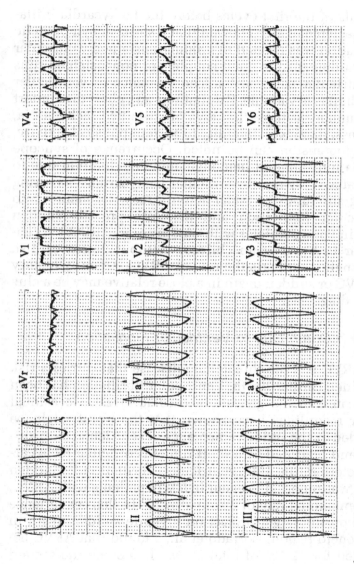

Figure 11. Twelve-lead electrocardiographic recording of sustained ventricular tachycardia in the setting of arrhythmogenic right ventricular cardiomyopathy. Note the left bundle branch block morphology associated to marked left axis deviation. Heart rate is 260 beats per minute.

intervals of the first cycles before the tachycardia initiation. Leclercq et al.[32] showed that a stronger sympathetic stimulation was needed to produce sustained ventricular tachycardias than to elicit couplets or nonsustained runs of ventricular tachycardia. The tolerance of ventricular arrhythmias is variable. Palpitations and chest discomfort are common features. In cases of sustained tachycardia, faintness, dizziness, inability to sustain physical activity, and hypotension can be noted. Occurrence of syncope may be indicative of hemodynamic deterioration due to high rates. Very rapid ventricular tachycardias occurring during strenuous physical activity may degenerate into ventricular fibrillation and therefore precede sudden death in young athletes with undiagnosed ARVC.[6,33] Ventricular tachycardia in children without patent cardiac abnormality supports the role of ARVC. A family history of ARVC or sudden death in a close relative may be a clue to the diagnosis.

Sudden Death Due to Ventricular Fibrillation

ARVC is a life-threatening disease that carries a risk of sudden cardiac death. Ventricular fibrillation has been implicated in the genesis of cardiac arrest. Occasional Holter recordings have shown that the event might be heralded by the sudden emergence of ventricular extrasystoles and preceded by a short run of ventricular tachycardia deteriorating into ventricular fibrillation.[33] Sudden death was reported to occur in 5% of patients with ARVC, with an annual rate of 2% to 3%.[34,35] In their experience based on the target project on juvenile sudden death in the Veneto region, Corrado et al.,[36] found that ARVC accounted for 12.5% of total cases, thus being the second most frequent cardiovascular cause of sudden death in the young (≤35 years), after coronary atherosclerosis, and the first cause of sudden death in the athletic population. On the contrary, sudden death due to ARVC seems to be anecdotal in American series.[37,38] As previously stated, whether these differences are accounted for by regional clustering or underdiagnosis of the disease remains a matter of uncertainty.

Unlike other causes of sudden death, such as coronary artery disease (congenital anomalies or atherosclerotic disease), in which prodroma in affected patients are seldom noticed, sudden death due to ARVC is rarely the first manifestation of the disease and preceding symptoms may have been present but overlooked because of their "benign" nature and the scarce awareness of the disease. Victims of sudden death have often been found retrospectively to have a family history of sudden death from heart disease or warning signs such as palpitations or syncope on exertion, electrocardiogram (ECG)-documented ventricular arrhythmias, and ECG abnormalities (inverted T waves in right precordial leads) that could have led to the identification of ARVC.[6] On the other hand, sudden cardiac death can always occur in patients with overt electrical disorders such as recurrent episodes of sustained ventricular tachycardia.[39-42] Progression of the disease is a possible cause. The role of drug-induced proarrhythmia, however, cannot be excluded, since Class I or Class III antiarrhythmic agents are commonly used in this setting. Documentation of very fast, polymorphic ventricular tachyarrhythmia may be a prelude to subsequent cardiac arrest.

Other Arrhythmic Events

Atrial arrhythmias have been reported in more than 20% of patients with ARVC.[43] The bases for supraventric-

ular disorders occurring in this setting are unclear. Myocardial abnormalities, hemodynamic factors, and sympathetic stimulation may play a role. All varieties can be
observed, ranging from atrial premature beats to sustained
arrhythmias such as atrial tachycardia, fibrillation, or flutter. Rarely, atrial tachyarrhythmias are the only events
present and constitute the first marker of the disease in
a young patient with an apparently normal heart.

Sick sinus syndrome is sometimes observed (Fig. 12).[5]
This is in accordance with the notion of sinus node
involvement put forward by pathologic reports. However,
increase in vagal tone may also account for bradycardia,
especially in athletes. Atrioventricular conduction disturbances are also seen[44,45]; these predominantly affect the
His-Purkinje system. Complete atrioventricular block can
ensue due to bilateral bundle branch block.[46] Conduction
disorders occur in the advanced stages of the disease,
in combination with cardiac dilatation and heart failure.
Interestingly atrioventricular conduction disturbances
can appear during antiarrhythmic drug therapy, thus un-
masking the underlying anomaly of the conduction system. Syncope, fatigue, and aggravation of the cardiovascular status are common features. Implantation of a cardiac
pacemaker, preferably dual-chamber, is indicated.

Heart Failure

Heart failure is a rare manifestation of ARVC. Prefer-
ential involvement of the right ventricle is a striking feature of ARVC and represents one of the most important
diagnostic criteria. In most cases, patients present with
isolated right heart failure, engorgement of the systemic
veins, and absence of pulmonary hypertension.[30] Fatigue

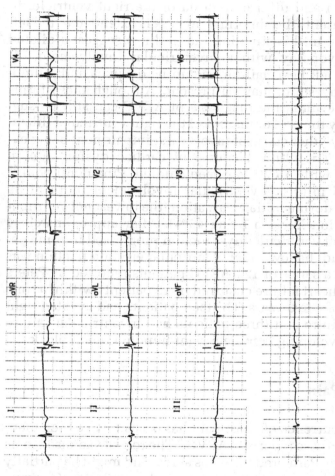

Figure 12. Twelve-lead electrocardiogram from a patient with extensive arrhythmogenic right ventricular cardiomyopathy. Sinus rhythm is disturbed by pauses ended by junctional escape beats. Sinus beats show incomplete right bundle branch block pattern and inverted T waves in leads I, II, aVL, and V_1 to V_6. Note at the end of QRS a tiny deflection (more clearly seen in leads V_4 to V_5) suggesting a postexcitation wave.

and exercise-induced disability are the dominant symptoms. Right heart failure is always associated with marked dilatation and diffuse akinesia of the right ventricle. In some patients the abnormal process is extended to the left ventricle. In this situation the findings suggest a dilated cardiomyopathy with a biventricular involvement.[30,47] Signs of left heart failure, including dyspnea and pulmonary congestion, may be present. Although these forms are misleading, the diagnosis of ARVC can still be suggested by the predominance of the right ventricular dilatation, any other cause of myocardial impairment being excluded. The clinical course of cardiac dysfunction in patients with ARVC has been studied. Pinamonti et al.[48] reported mild left ventricular involvement in 14 of 39 patients during initial evaluation (the lowest left ventricular ejection fraction being 45%). After approximately 4 years, left ventricular dysfunction progressed in some patients and the lowest left ventricular ejection fraction was 24%. In a series of 121 ARVC patients reported by Peters et al.,[30] heart failure occurred in 16 patients within a time course of 4 to 8 years. Thirteen patients had isolated right heart failure and three patients had biventricular failure after developing complete right bundle branch block.

Chest Pain

Occurrence of chest pain has occasionally been mentioned in case reports of ARVC.[5] The role of exercise seems to be rare. Pain predominates at rest and might be partially relieved by vasodilative drugs such as nitrates. Obstruction of distal coronary vessels embedded in fatty tissue or myocardium has been demonstrated in pathologic studies.[49] This provides a potential substrate for myocardial ischemia. The implication of vasospasms is invoked but requires further elucidation.

Latent Forms

The notion of latent forms of ARVC is well accepted. Patients who carry the disease can remain free of symptoms. As previously mentioned, the actual prevalence of latent forms of ARVC is unknown. These silent cases are likely to occur among relatives of patients with familial ARVC. Whether the absence of symptoms can be indefinite or rather transient and followed by overt ARVC is uncertain. No consistent follow-up data dealing with this category of subjects are available, any related study being difficult to perform. In asymptomatic patients, presence of the disease can be documented by noninvasive tests, indicating that the arrhythmogenic substrate is present but silent. These patients may have electrocardiographic signs of ARVC and late potentials revealed by signal averaging (see further). The value of positive tests in screening asymptomatic family members of patients with a history of sudden death requires further investigation. Progress in genetics should be a determinant for detecting latent forms of ARVC and better defining the phenotypic patterns of the disease.

Diagnostic Tools

Physical Examination

Although the physical examination in patients with ARVC is usually unremarkable, a split first or second heart sound, a systolic murmur in the tricuspid area, or a third or fourth heart sound occasionally may be present.[5] In young patients there may be prominence of the left precordium consistent with right ventricular enlargement. Presence of right ventricular insufficiency in the absence of significant valvular disease may be suggestive of ARVC. However, no sign is specific. In many cases physical examination is quite normal, which of course should not preclude the eventuality of ARVC.

Chest X-Ray

In the majority of patients, chest x-ray is normal. However, a moderate cardiac enlargement without pulmonary vascular redistribution may be present in some patients. The heart is then globular in configuration (Fig. 13). Concomitant right atrial dilatation is sometimes noted. In competitive athletes this cardiomegaly is likely to be wrongly attributed to training. The cardiothoracic index is less than 0.6 in most cases.[16]

ECG in Sinus Rhythm

The ECG is a major tool for the diagnosis of ARVC. The electrocardiographic abnormalities are commonly the first markers of the underlying disease. In combination with clinical features, their presence strongly supports the notion of ARVC. The magnitude of the changes, however, is highly variable and the electrocardiographic patterns bear different diagnostic values. The following abnormalities have been reported in patients with suspected ARVC:

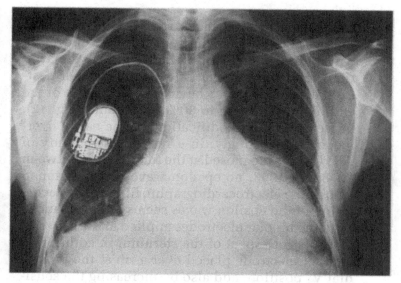

Figure 13. Chest x-ray obtained from a patient with a severe form of arrhythmogenic right ventricular cardiomyopathy. The cardiac silhouette is enlarged and globular in configuration. This is accounted for by a marked dilatation of the right cardiac cavities. On the other hand, the size of the left ventricle was normal at echocardiography. Note that the patient has a cardiac pacemaker because of previous occurrence of complete atrioventricular block.

1. Prolonged QRS duration ≥110 ms in lead V_1 was reported to carry a sensitivity of 55% and a specificity of 100% in series of patients whose initial manifestation was mostly sustained ventricular tachycardia. Like other features, prevalence figures are only drawn from overt forms of the disease. They are likely to be different in the various clinical subsets. Generally, the QRS duration is more prolonged in lead V_1 as compared to leads I and V_6.[50] Complete or incomplete right bundle branch block are also common findings and may

result from parietal block rather than disease of the right bundle branch per se (Figs. 12 and 14).[46]

2. An abnormal deflection resulting from delayed right ventricular activation (epsilon wave or post-excitation wave)[4] may be noticed at the end of the QRS complex in up to 30% of patients (Fig. 12). In fact, this tiny modification can be easily overlooked. Interestingly, in a retrospective study of ARVC cases diagnosed at the Mayo Clinic between 1978 and 1993, no epsilon wave was mentioned among the electrocardiographic findings.[34] Recognition of the epsilon waves seems to be enhanced by using bipolar electrodes applied at the superior and inferior aspect of the sternum, in addition to another electrode placed over a rib at the precordial V_4 position, and also by increasing the sensitivity twofold.[5]

3. Low-voltage QRS amplitude (defined as QRS amplitude <5 mm in leads I, II, and III or <10 mm in precordial leads) may indicate a widespread myocardial process.[51]

4. T wave inversion in right precordial leads is frequently encountered (about 60% of patients with T wave abnormalities in leads V_1 through V_3 and up to 80% in leads V_1 and V_2) and remains the most suggestive indicator of ARVC.[5] More diffuse patterns can be seen with T wave anomalies also present in the inferior leads. Inverted T waves have an ischemic pattern with both limbs showing almost similar slopes (Figs. 7, 8, 12, 14, and 15). This should be differentiated from nonspecific repolarization abnormalities associated with right bundle branch block. The significance of ST-segment elevation in right precordial leads for the

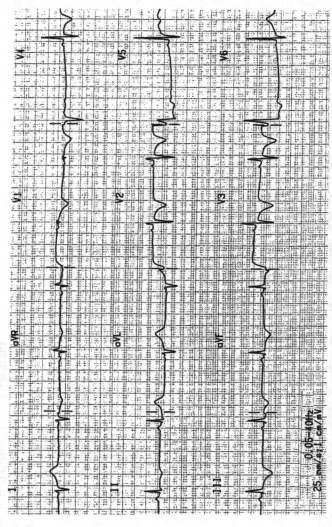

Figure 14. Twelve-lead electrocardiographic recording in a patient with extensive arrhythmogenic right ventricular cardiomyopathy. The QRS complexes in sinus rhythm exhibit incomplete right bundle branch block morphology and right axis deviation. T wave inversion is seen in leads V_1 to V_5 and in the inferior leads.

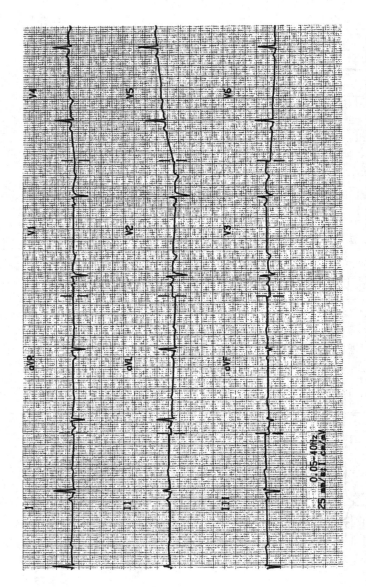

Figure 15. Twelve-lead electrocardiogram obtained during sinus rhythm from a patient with arrhythmogenic right ventricular cardiomyopathy. Note T wave inversion in leads V_1 to V_5. QRS frontal axis is normal. No conduction disturbance is apparent.

diagnosis of ARVC is uncertain,[52] except for the dynamic changes recorded during exercise (see further). Interestingly, occurrence of ST-segment elevation following administration of antiarrhythmics is occasionally observed.

5. Increased QT dispersion has been noted in patients with ARVC compared to control subjects. However, the degree of dispersion was not related to the severity of symptoms, nor was it influenced by antiarrhythmic treatment with sotalol.[53] The significance of QT dispersion per se is controversial and its clinical relevance is currently contested.

In a follow-up study on 20 patients with symptomatic ARVC,[51] electrocardiographic abnormalities were present in 90% of patients. However, no correlation was found between abnormalities on the initial 12-lead ECG and the echocardiographic extent and location of the right ventricular involvement. Serial electrocardiographic recordings over a 71-month follow-up period did not provide information regarding anatomical progression of the disease. On the other hand, Jaoude et al.[54] reported a normal ECG in up to 40% of their patients referred for arrhythmic events resulting from ARVC. During a 9.5-year follow-up, electrocardiographic changes (negative T waves, new left axis deviation, QRS enlargement, right atrial hypertrophy, and atrial fibrillation) were observed in 56% of the patients studied, and were correlated to the length of follow-up after the initial symptom.

Exercise Stress Test

The exercise stress test is an important diagnostic tool and must be performed in every case of ARVC. This is

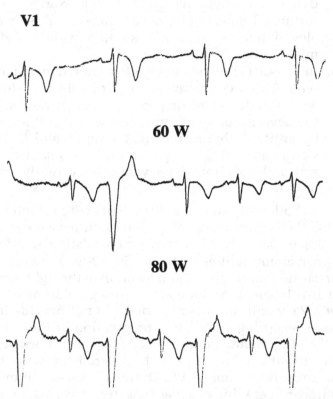

Figure 16. Exercise stress test performed in a patient suffering from arrhythmogenic right ventricular cardiomyopathy-related ventricular arrhythmias. During exercise, isolated ventricular premature beats appear, followed by ventricular bigeminy.

based on the notion that ARVC-related arrhythmias are often triggered by exercise and show adrenergic tone dependency. Among cardiomyopathies, ARVC is the one that is most likely to develop ventricular rhythm disorders during exertion (Fig. 16). In a young adult without apparent heart disease, such a response leads one to suggest the possibility of ARVC. In this setting, however, the findings during stress test are not unequivocal. The exercise stress test reportedly exacerbates ventricular arrhythmias in approximately half of the patients with ARVC.[55] The number of ventricular premature beats can rise markedly with adjunction of couplets, salvos, or possibly deterioration into sustained ventricular tachycardia or ventricular fibrillation. The aggravation of the arrhythmic events is associated with increasingly high levels of exercise. Other patients experience no worsening of ventricular arrhythmias during exercise. This should not be misinterpreted and used in support of a benign condition. Lack of proarrhythmic response during exercise does not exclude ARVC.[55]

In addition to ventricular arrhythmias, the exercise stress test performed in patients with ARVC may induce repolarization abnormalities. Local or diffuse wall motion alterations in patients with ARVC may provoke ST-segment elevation in response to exercise. Toyofuku et al.[56] observed exercise-induced ST-segment elevation of more than 0.1 mV in 65% of their patients with ARVC. This finding was more frequently noted in right precordial leads. Since exercise-induced ST-segment elevation is a rare phenomenon in normal subjects and noninvasive imaging techniques such as echocardiography and radionuclide angiography cannot always detect the abnormal morphology of the right ventricle, this observation may be of use for identifying patients with ARVC.

Signal-Averaged ECG

The fibrofatty replacement characteristic of ARVC interrupts the electrical continuity of myocardial fibers, which accounts for conduction delay. In the abnormal area, late depolarization may persist after the end of the complex QRS because of slow conduction. This low-voltage activity assumedly represents a potential source of ventricular reexcitation. As previously mentioned, it can occasionally be seen on the ECG accounting for the so-called epsilon wave. In this view the techniques of amplification and signal averaging are required to detect such late potentials that would be otherwise unidentified (Fig. 17). Currently, the signal-averaged ECG is always performed in the assessment of patients with suspected ARVC.

Mehta et al.[57] found abnormal signal-averaged ECGs, using time domain analysis, in 90% of patients with ARVC and ventricular tachycardia of right ventricular origin. There was a strong correlation between all signal-averaged ECG parameters and right ventricular cavity dimensions. Nava et al.[58] determined the sensitivity, specificity, and predictive value of abnormal signal-averaged ECGs in 138 patients with different degrees of ARVC (minor, moderate, and extensive) compared to 146 healthy subjects. The signal-averaged ECG had an overall sensitivity of 57%, a specificity of 95%, and a positive predictive value of 92%. A closer correlation was noted with the extent of disease than with the presence of ventricular arrhythmias: late potentials were present in 94.4% of patients with the extensive form of the disease, in 77.7% of patients with the moderate form, and only in 31.8% of patients with the minor form. With regard to different types of arrhythmias, there was a greater percentage of patients with ventricular fibrillation or sustained ventricular tachycardia who had abnormal signal-averaged ECGs (71% and 72%, respectively), and this percentage rose to 94.4% in the subgroup of patients with ventricular tachycardia of superior axis.

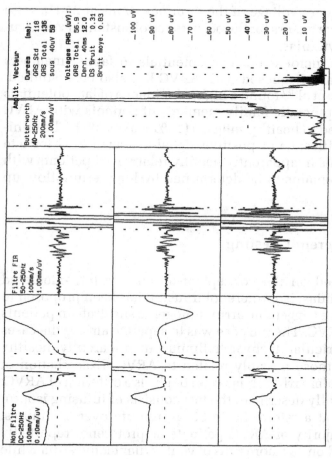

Figure 17. Signal-averaged electrocardiogram recorded from a patient with arrhythmogenic right ventricular cardiomyopathy. Amplified electrograms in leads X, Y, and Z are shown in the left and middle panels. After summation and averaging, the filtered QRS exhibits late potentials (in black) at the end of the ventriculogram.

Turini et al.[59] found that low right ventricular ejection fraction was the most powerful predictor of late potentials. Both a right ventricular ejection fraction ≤0.5 and the root mean square voltage of the terminal 40 ms at 25 Hz were predictive factors for the occurrence of sustained ventricular arrhythmias.

The incidence of late potentials in family members of patients diagnosed with ARVC has also been studied. Hermida et al.[60] found a higher incidence of late potentials in asymptomatic family members of patients with ARVC compared to healthy subjects (16% versus 3%). The clinical significance of positive signal-averaged ECG for late potentials in apparently healthy relatives of patients with ARVC remains to be determined by long-term follow-up studies.

Isoproterenol Testing

Based on the concept of adrenergic tone-mediated arrhythmias, isoproterenol infusion has been proposed to unmask a triggerable arrhythmogenic substrate in patients with ARVC. The purpose was to separate among the cases of ventricular tachyarrhythmias in apparently healthy people those possibly related to ARVC. Exacerbation of ventricular arrhythmias was sought as a criterion of ARVC. As initially described, the test consists of infusing isoproterenol at a rate of 20 to 30 μg/minute over 3 minutes. In a majority of ARVC patients isoproterenol reportedly induced one or more runs of ventricular tachycardia while sustained tachyarrhythmias occurred in less than one third of subjects.[61] Most episodes were polymorphic, the predominant morphology being that of left bundle branch block. The test appears to be reproducible. In control subjects with or without ventricular premature beats, the response to isoproterenol was unremarkable. Thus, isoproterenol infusion seems to be highly sensitive for the diagnosis of ARVC; however, it should be used with caution in patients with suspected coronary artery disease. Interestingly, the test may be positive in the absence of late potentials. Despite these convincing findings, use of isoproterenol infusion in ARVC patients remains marginal as a first-intent screening test. No subsequent study has been performed to further elucidate the role of isoproterenol testing in ARVC.

Electrophysiologic Study

The ability to induce and terminate ventricular tachycardias related to ARVC by programmed ventricular stimulation supports a reentrant mechanism (Fig. 18). Electrophysiologic testing aims to provide evidence for an arrhythmogenic substrate, to define the electrophysiologic characteristics of the arrhythmia, and, in selected cases, to guide therapy. However, the value of programmed electrical stimulation to predict occurrence of spontaneous ventricular arrhythmias is quite low. In order to improve the sensitivity of the test, pacing should be performed at more than one right ventricular site and, in some cases, from the left ventricle, using different basic cycle lengths, one to three extrastimuli, and bursts. In patients with mild forms of ARVC, DiBiase et al.[62] found that programmed stimulation induced ventricular tachycardia mainly in the subgroup with spontaneous sustained ventricular tachycardia. Only 13% of patients with repetitive ventricular ectopies had inducible sustained tachyarrhythmias. Occasionally, induction of sustained ventricular tachycardia

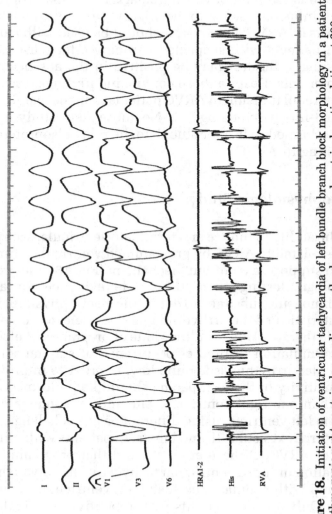

Figure 18. Initiation of ventricular tachycardia of left bundle branch block morphology in a patient with arrhythmogenic right ventricular cardiomyopathy, by programmed ventricular stimulation at 600-ms cycle length with three extrastimuli. Surface leads I, II, V_1, V_3, and V_6 are shown, along with intracardiac electrograms from the high right atrium (HRA), the His bundle (HBE), and the right ventricular apex (RVA). Note the atrioventricular dissociation during tachycardia.

may require administration of isoproterenol.[61] Similarly, Peters and Reil[63] reported inducible ventricular tachycardia in 90% of patients with spontaneous sustained tachycardia episodes. In this study, sustained ventricular tachycardia was noninducible in all patients with nonsustained attacks and ventricular ectopies and in 30% of patients with previous cardiac arrest even after isoproterenol infusion. It is noteworthy that ventricular fibrillation is sometimes initiated by programmed stimulation, but its prognostic value is so far unclear.[64] In cardiac arrest survivors, however, such a response to electrophysiologic testing is more likely to be clinically relevant. Use of isoproterenol infusion may improve the sensitivity of programmed electrical stimulation in ARVC patients.

Electrophysiologic study can shed some insight into the arrhythmogenic area. The vast majority of ventricular tachycardias in patients with ARVC occur at sites with delayed, fractionated, and low-voltage electrograms during sinus rhythm. These diastolic potentials are tiny deflections recorded outside the QRS complex and exhibiting rate-dependent properties.[65] However, abnormal electrograms may be widespread in the right ventricle, and their predictive value to determine the site of origin of ventricular tachycardia is poor.

Pace mapping techniques[66] suggest that ventricular tachycardia in ARVC shares many of the characteristics seen in post myocardial infarction patients. Electrical stimulation at the site of diastolic potentials may result in a long time interval between the electrical stimulus and the ventricular response due to delayed emergence of the impulse from the slow conduction area (Fig. 19). During tachycardia entrainment may ensue, which is of further help for delineating the ablation target.

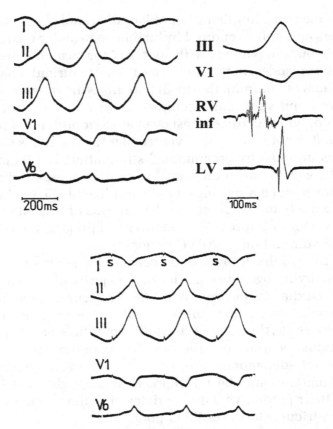

Figure 19. Electrophysiologic findings in a patient with arrhythmogenic right ventricular cardiomyopathy-related ventricular tachycardia. During tachycardia, the QRS complexes show left bundle branch block morphology and right axis deviation (top). Heart rate is 200 beats per minute. Endocardial mapping demonstrates early ventricular activation of the right ventricular infundibulum (RV inf) with splitting of the local electrogram. There is also a presystolic potential preceding the onset of QRS by 40 ms. Electrical stimulation at this site produces paced beats similar to the tachycardia beats (bottom). LV = left ventricle; s = stimulus artifact.

Finally, programmed electrical stimulation has also been shown to induce atrial tachyarrhythmias in patients with ARVC.[67] The significance of this phenomenon is under debate. It is unclear whether such a response implies involvement of the atrial myocardium in the setting of a diffuse process.

Echocardiographic Findings

Echocardiographic studies may show localized abnormalities of the right heart cavities, increased thickness of the moderator band, and trabeculations of the right ventricular apex. There may be obvious irregular dilatation of the outflow tract with an increased right ventricle/left ventricle ratio.[68] However, in minor forms, the abnormality is difficult to detect. The structural changes in most cases of ARVC are moderate.[69] They can be recognized only if systematically sought, especially by measuring diameters at several strategic points of the right ventricle. These measurements should be compared with normal values, according to a protocol by Foale et al.[70]

Morphologic abnormalities found on two-dimensional echocardiography include dilatation of the right ventricle, thin ventricular wall with akinetic areas, presence of aneurysms during diastole, and dyskinetic areas in the inferobasal region, particularly specific when observed below the tricuspid valve (Fig. 20). Parasternal views with the patients lying on the right lateral should be performed systematically when ARVC is suspected. With the subcostal approach it is possible to see the free wall of the right ventricle in the two-dimensional mode and on time motion echocardiography. Rotating the probe 90 degrees enables one to visualize the long axis of the

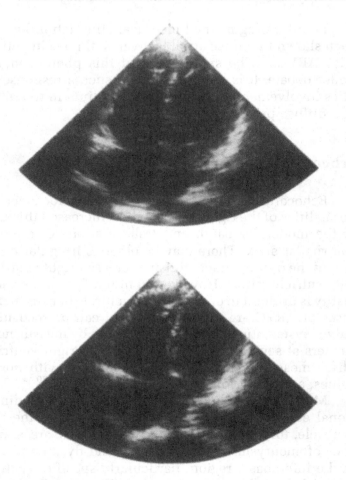

Figure 20. Top: modified apical four-chamber echocardiogram obtained from a patient with extensive arrhythmogenic right ventricular cardiomyopathy showing severely dilated right cavities and a right-to-left ventricular ratio greater than 1. Bottom: apical four-chamber echocardiogram from a different patient demonstrating moderately enlarged right ventricle with a dyskinetic area at its apex.

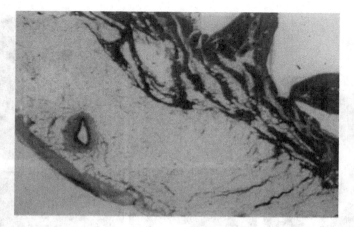

Figure 3

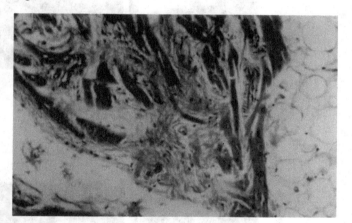

Figure 4

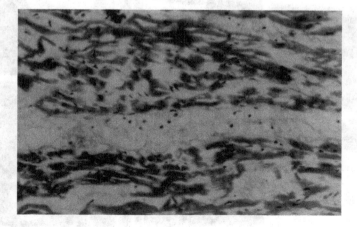

Figure 5

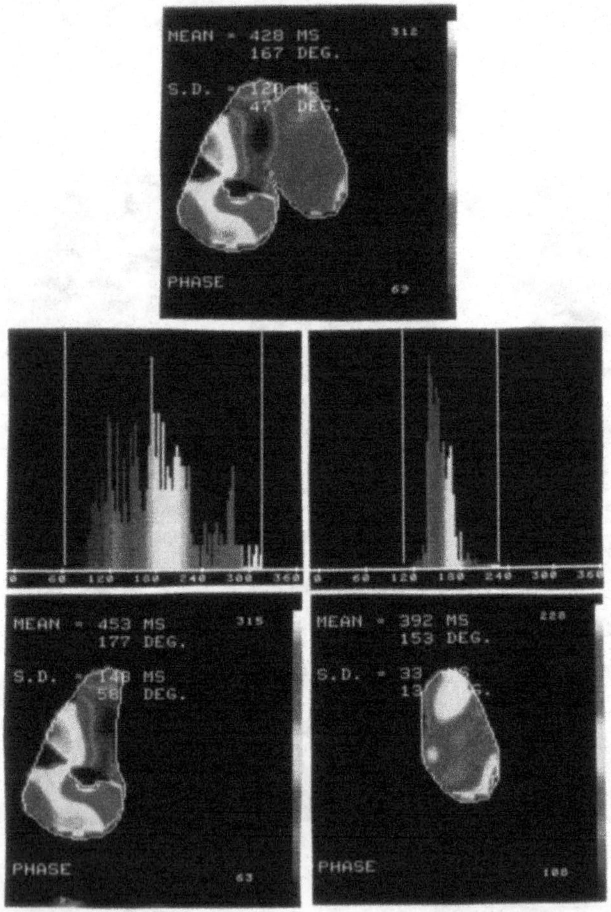

Figure 22

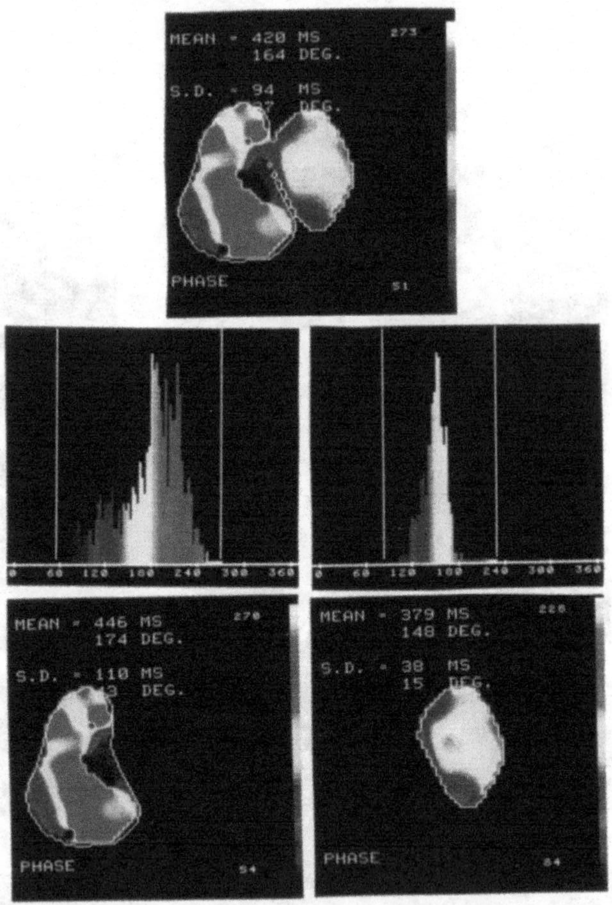

Figure 23

right ventricle, which is useful for studying the infundibulum and pulmonary artery. Particular attention must be paid to tricuspid valve prolapse and regurgitation in the severe forms of the disease, as well as mitral valve prolapse, which has been recently recognized as a condition frequently associated with ARVC.[71] Contrast echocardiography using injections of saline may help to evaluate right ventricular regional or global function. Contrast echocardiography may better outline the right ventricle to allow measurement of the right ventricular volume. Transesophageal echocardiography may be more sensitive than a transthoracic approach in detecting wall motion abnormalities. Three-dimensional echocardiography, particularly combined with a transesophageal approach, is being investigated to enhance the diagnostic accuracy of this technique.[72]

Echocardiography can also detect involvement of the left ventricle. Usually the left ventricular cavity is unremarkable and the ejection fraction is within the normal range. The coexistence of right ventricular alteration and normal left ventricle in a patient with ventricular tachycardia of left bundle branch block configuration is actually suggestive of ARVD. However, as previously stated, the left ventricle occasionally exhibits segmental or diffuse dyskinesia, dilatation, and depressed function. These findings may render the diagnosis of ARVC more difficult.

As a whole, two-dimensional echocardiography is an essential tool for the early diagnosis of ARVC. Definite right ventricular abnormalities at echocardiography are invaluable. Conversely, a negative test does not preclude the diagnosis of ARVC. Echocardiography must be included in any investigation undertaken to detect the familial incidence of the disease.

Endomyocardial Biopsy

In most cases, confirmation of the diagnosis by endomyocardial biopsy is not required. This technique may be useful to demonstrate the typical, highly diagnostic, histologic abnormalities of ARVC provided the biopsy is directed to the affected areas. However, the endomyocardial biopsy provides samples from the subendocardium and the subendocardial picture does not necessarily reflect the transmural picture.[73] The exclusive presence of fibrotic specimens in ARVC patients is not surprising. In the fibrofatty variant of ARVC, fibrous tissue tends to be prevalently distributed within the subendocardial area, whereas fatty tissue predominates in the midepicardial or subepicardial layers. Because ARVC is a focal disease, the biopsy may not be a sensitive tool for the degree of fibrous and fatty infiltration. On the other hand, one should keep in mind that, considering the thin and atrophic right ventricular walls of these patients, this technique is an invasive procedure associated with the potential risk of perforation and cardiac tamponade. Therefore, such procedure should be restricted to very controversial cases and directed to the affected areas as demonstrated by imaging techniques. Otherwise, sensitivity of this test is low because, for reasons of safety, samples are usually taken from the septum, a region not commonly involved with the disease.

Right Contrast Ventriculography

Cineangiographic investigation is currently used to evaluate the morphologic and functional status of cardiac cavities and parietal walls. Cardiomegaly, deep fissures, margin changes, localized akinetic or dyskinetic bulges, out-pouchings, dilatation of the right ventricular outflow tract, and slow dye evacuation are the most frequently reported angiocardiographic parameters associated with the fibrofatty replacement in the right ventricle of patients diagnosed with ARVC (Fig. 21).[74,75] Daliento et al.[76] found that transversally arranged hypertrophic trabeculae, separated by deep fissures and located in the apical region distal to the moderator band, were associated with the highest probability of ARVC. Posterior subtricuspid and infundibular wall bulgings were the other independent diagnostic variables for ARVC. In this study, coexistence of these signs was associated with 87.5% sensitivity and 96% specificity. However, right ventricular angiographic abnormalities are often difficult to assess because of the complex geometry of this chamber. This is particularly true for right ventricular enlargement appraisal, despite the availability of validated measurement methods. It is noteworthy that increase in right ventricular volume is a frequent feature in patients with ARVC, whereas localized bulgings or out-pouchings are manifestations of the disease in only a small percentage of these patients. Right ventricular angiography is not necessarily performed in any patient with suspected ARVC. In asymptomatic patients with suggestive echocardiographic findings, further evidence can be provided by other noninvasive imaging modalities. On the other hand, right ventricular angiography is usually included in the assessment of patients presenting with malignant ventricular arrhythmias of uncertain origin. In suspected cases angiography may be combined with myocardial biopsies.

Radionuclide Angiography and Computed Tomography

Radionuclide angiography is another useful diagnostic tool that may overcome the limitations of contrast ven-

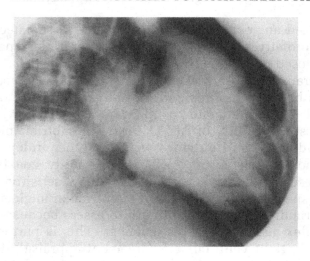

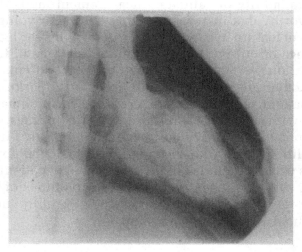

Figure 21. Right contrast ventriculography performed from the right atrium (right anterior oblique view) in a patient with advanced form of arrhythmogenic right ventricular cardiomyopathy. Note deep fissures and the marked right ventricular dilatation compared to left ventricle (bottom).

triculography. Analysis of right ventricular segmental wall motion is complex because of the particular morphology and trabeculations of the right ventricle, the presence of frequent premature beats during angiography, and the difficulty of obtaining a technically adequate angiogram. Furthermore, the reproducibility of contrast ventriculography is not optimal.[75] Radionuclide angiography permits mathematical fitting of the pixel ventricular curve by means of Fourier analysis. This analysis has been demonstrated to be of value in detection of right and left wall motion abnormalities and aneurysms.[77,78] These abnormalities reflect on the distribution histogram that depicts a typical double peak morphology or late regional phase distribution, as opposed to the single peak homogeneous phase distribution histogram observed in normal subjects. In a prospective study on patients with ventricular tachycardia originating from the right ventricle, Le Guludec et al.[79] compared contrast and radionuclide angiography for the diagnosis of ARVC. The sensitivity of the latter technique was 94.3%, the specificity 90%, and the positive and negative predictive values were 96% and 85.7%, respectively. Agreement between the two techniques for the location of wall motion abnormalities was 60% for the apex, 76% for the outflow tract, 82% for the inferior wall, and 74% for the free wall. The reproducibility of the technique (96.2%) also makes it possible to follow the progression of right ventricular wall motion abnormalities. Reliable simultaneous analysis of the left ventricle is of importance to detect cases of ARVC with left ventricular involvement. Radionuclide angiography belongs to the first-intent investigations that are performed to identify ARVC patients, and usually replaces invasive ventriculography.

Given the complex morphology of the right ventricle and the difficulty of tricuspid annulus delineation on planar study, however, a tomographic method might be more helpful. Gated blood pool single-photon emission tomography (GBP-SPECT) has been demonstrated to be more accurate than planar studies for right volume determination but also for detection of left ventricular wall motion abnormalities. Casset-Senon et al.[80] found the following abnormalities on GBP-SPECT in 18 patients with ARVC: significantly decreased right ventricular ejection fraction, right ventricle dilatation, nonsynchronized contraction of the ventricles, increased right ventricular contraction dispersion, presence of right ventricular wall motion disorders and/or phase delays, and occasional left ventricular abnormalities (Figs. 22 and 23). The same authors proposed a scoring system with these criteria to diagnose ARVC. In addition, multiharmonic and factor analysis can be used to enhance the diagnostic capabilities[81] (third harmonic Fourier analysis for detecting outflow tract and inferior wall motion abnormalities, and factor analysis for the right ventricular apex).

[123]I-Meta-Iodobenzylguanidine Scintigraphy

In patients with ARVC, regional abnormalities of sympathetic innervation are frequent and can be demonstrated by ^{123}I-meta-iodobenzylguanidine (^{123}I-MIBG) scintigraphy. Wichter et al.[29] observed a regional reduction in ^{123}I-MIBG uptake in 40 of 48 patients with ARVC that they studied with this technique, whereas the tracer distribution was found to be homogenous in all control subjects. Sympathetic denervation appears to be the underlying mechanism of reduced ^{123}I-MIBG uptake. Therefore, in

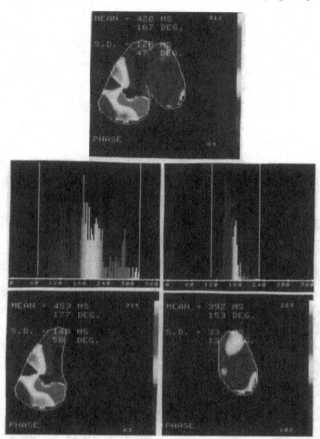

Figure 22. Gated blood pool tomographic data (short axis) obtained from a patient diagnosed with arrhythmogenic right ventricular cardiomyopathy with no left ventricular involvement. Top: phase analysis of the right and left ventricles showing significant contraction delay in the right ventricle relative to the left ventricle. Middle: phase histograms of the right ventricle (left) and the left ventricle (right). The histogram corresponding to the left ventricle shows a homogeneous distribution of contraction phases, whereas the right ventricular histogram is much more dispersed due to heterogeneity of contraction. Bottom: phase dispersion more pronounced in the right ventricle (left) as compared to the left ventricle (right), expressed as mean phase and phase standard deviation. A color version of this image can be found on the color insert.

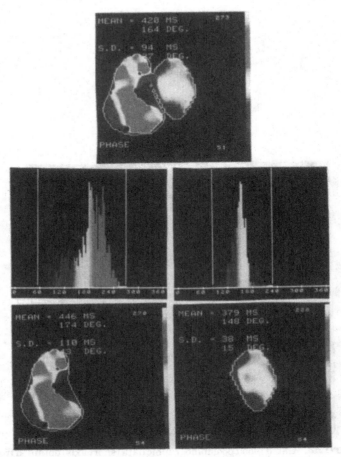

Figure 23. Gated blood pool tomographic data (short axis) in a case of arrhythmogenic right ventricular cardiomyopathy. The significance of the upper, middle, and lower panels is similar to that depicted in Figure 22. Compared to the left ventricle, the right ventricle exhibits marked contraction delay and heterogeneity of contraction with more accentuated phase dispersion. A color version of this image can be found on the color insert.

patients with ARVC, the noninvasive detection of localized sympathetic denervation by ^{123}I-MIBG imaging may
have implications for the early diagnosis of the disease.

Magnetic Resonance Imaging

Magnetic resonance imaging (MRI) is an emerging
noninvasive technique that provides cardiac images with
a high spatial resolution and enables an accurate morpho-
functional assessment of the right ventricle and detection
of features characteristic of ARVC such as trabecular disar-
ray, bulges, and aneurysms.[82] The spin echo technique is
used to identify areas of fatty replacement (hyperintensity)
(Fig. 24).[83] Therefore, the MRI is the only noninvasive
tool to provide information on tissue composition. The
identification of abnormal areas may be helpful to guide
the cardiac electrophysiologist in mapping ventricular arrhythmias. Given that fatty tissue may be present to a
varying extent in patients who do not have ARVC, recording hyperintensity zones on MRI must be interpreted
with caution. Cine-MRI using gradient echo sequences
improves temporal resolution sufficiently to identify end-
systole and end-diastole, thereby enabling measurements
of global and regional right and left ventricular function.[83]
Some have reported that MRI imaging may detect abnormalities that were not previously visualized by echocardiography or angiography in patients with ARVC.[84] However, the sensitivity of this technique is too low and its
potential for diagnosing concealed forms of ARVC remains
controversial. Further studies are needed to define the
actual role of MRI in the diagnostic approach to ARVC.

Genetics

A family history of ARVC is present in 30% to 50%
of ARVC patients.[18-21] The most common form of transmis-

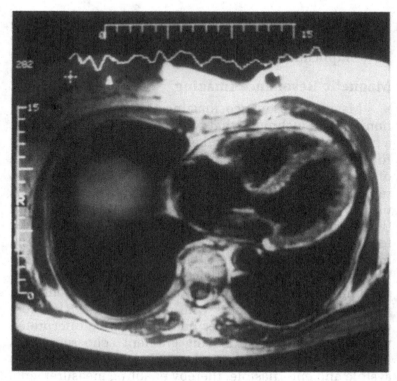

Figure 24. Magnetic resonance imaging in a case of right ventricular dysplasia. Axial spin-echo image shows thin and hyperintense wall of the right ventricle. High signal intensity, presumably due to fatty infiltration, extends from pericardial layer to endocardium.

sion is autosomal dominant with incomplete penetrance and variable expression, which accounts for the appearance of minor forms of the disease. An autosomal recessive pattern has also been reported. Although the gene has not been identified, linkage analysis in the dominant form has located the genetic abnormality on chromosomes 1 (1q42-q43), 2 (2q32.1-q32.2), and 14 with two loci in close proximity (14q23-q24 and 14q12-q22).[85-88] The autosomal recessive syndromic variant of ARVD has been linked to a locus on chromosome 17 (17q21) within the gene encoding a keratin.[89] This latter form, characteristically associated with epidermal abnormalities such as palmoplantar keratosis and woolly hair, has been reported from the island of Naxos in Greece. In this condition, signs of the disease are more severe and penetrance in family members is 90%. Some families are not linked to these loci, which suggests further genetic heterogeneity. The genetic basis of ARVC is still under investigation. Further advances will facilitate recognition of variant phenotypes of the disease.

Clinical Approach to ARVC

As previously mentioned, the incidence of ARVC was found to be significantly different in Europe than in North America. The bases for the higher incidence of the disease in northern Italy compared to North America remain to be elucidated.

In a majority of cases, the identification of ARVC is a matter of debate and carries variable degrees of uncertainty. The presence of the disease is considered possible or probable without any definite evidence of specific right ventricular abnormalities. Despite a remarkable development of the investigation tools, the diagnosis of ARVC remains a clinical challenge in patients with minimal right ventricular changes at echocardiographic or angiographic examination. Although endomyocardial biopsy has the potential to provide in vivo demonstration of fibrofatty infiltration of the heart, samples are usually taken, for safety reasons, from the septum, an area not commonly involved with the disease.[73] Evidence for ARVC is indirect and can result from different sources. The electrocardiographic alterations are commonly a starting point combining ventricular arrhythmias and repolarization abnormalities in the right precordial leads. Signal-averaged ECG may detect late potentials in the vast majority of patients with widespread disease but is negative in a significant number of focal forms. Exacerbation of ventricular rhythm disorders following exercise or isoprenaline infusion supports the notion of ARVC; however, this response is by no means specific. Radionuclide angiography is currently a preferred method to assess size and wall motion anomalies of the right ventricle, and should be included in any diagnostic approach to the disease. MRI appears to be promising in the evaluation of the right ventricular changes, but normal range limits for right ventricular volumes and regional function are under debate. In the same view, the recognition of fatty deposits lacks accuracy, and the distinction between normal and abnormal aspects remains controversial. Furthermore, the relevant studies are of limited size and there is considerable heterogeneity of findings. Currently, sensitivity and specificity of MRI still need to be defined. At the other end of the disease's spectrum, there are those forms exhibiting diffuse alterations extended to the left ventricle. Prominent right ventricular dilatation should lead the diagnostic tools toward the search for ARVC. In this setting MRI may be of particular interest by detecting increased adipose tissue within the ventricular myocardium.

Because of these difficulties, a set of diagnostic criteria for ARVC was recently proposed by the task force of the Working Group on Myocardial and Pericardial Diseases of the European Society of Cardiology and the Scientific Council of Cardiomyopathies of the International Society and Federation of Cardiology.[90] "Major" and "minor" criteria were distinguished (Table 1). According to this consensus, the diagnosis of ARVC can be made if there is a combination of two major criteria, one major plus two minor criteria, or four minor criteria. A clinical validation of the proposed criteria on large series of patients is not presently available; however, this stepwise approach should enhance the diagnostic capabilities and help homogenize the bases of ARVC identification.

Differential Diagnosis

Right Ventricular Outflow Tract Tachycardia

Differentiation between ARVC and the so-called right ventricular outflow tract tachycardias, a usually benign and nonfamilial condition, is a practical problem. Patients present with paroxysms of tachyarrhythmias with left bundle branch block morphology. Long-term outcome is favorable with drug therapy. Radiofrequency catheter ablation can be performed successfully to treat refractory forms. Moreover, whether the right ventricular outflow tract tachycardia is a variant of ARVC is still debated.[91] The context may help differentiate this type of arrhythmia from true ARVC. For instance, as opposed to ARVC, ECG recordings in sinus rhythm do not show persisting repolarization abnormalities and ventricular premature beats are often absent. Furthermore, adrenergic tone dependency is not necessarily associated with the occurrence of attacks. In some cases modern imaging techniques appear to detect anomalies indicative of ARVC.[91] However one must take into account the uncertainties of all diagnostic tools, particularly when used to detect localized forms of

Table 1

Criteria for Diagnosis of Arrhythmogenic Right Ventricular Cardiomyopathy

I.   Global and/or regional dysfunction and structural alteration

MAJOR   Severe dilatation and reduction of right ventricular ejection fraction with no (or only mild) left ventricular impairment

Localized right ventricular aneurysms (akinetic or dyskinetic areas with diastolic bulging)

Severe segmental dilatation of the right ventricle

MINOR   Mild global right ventricular dilatation and/or ejection fraction reduction with normal left ventricle

II.   Tissue characterization of walls

MAJOR   Fibrofatty replacement of myocardium on endomyocardial biopsy

III.   Repolarization abnormalities

MINOR   Inverted T waves in right precordial leads (V_2 and V_3) (people older than 12 years; in the absence of right bundle branch block)

IV.   Depolarization/conduction abnormalities

MAJOR   Epsilon waves or localized prolongation (>110 ms) of the QRS complex in right precordial leads (V_1-V_3)

MINOR   Late potentials (signal-averaged ECG)

V.   Arrhythmias

MINOR   Left bundle branch block type ventricular tachycardia (sustained and nonsustained) (ECG, Holter, exercise testing)

Frequent ventricular extrasystoles (>1000/24 h) (Holter)

VI.   Family history

MAJOR   Familial disease confirmed at necropsy or surgery

MINOR   Family history of premature sudden death (<35 years) due to suspected right ventricular dysplasia

Family history (clinical diagnosis based on present criteria)

ARVC. The role of the so-called right ventricular outflow tract tachycardia as a clinical presentation of ARVC remains to be established.

Uhl's Disease

Another matter of discussion is Uhl's disease.[55] In this setting, aplasia of the right ventricular wall consists of apposition of endocardium and epicardium without intervening muscular fibers. This anomaly is considered to be congenital, due to a disontogenetic process.[2,7] There is no fat or inflammatory reaction in the myocardium. No family history is noted. Whereas ARVC occurs predominantly in males, there is no such gender difference in Uhl's anomaly. Age at presentation is also different. Uhl's anomaly is identified in infants or during childhood, while the first manifestations of ARVC usually affect adolescents or adults. The major clinical manifestation of Uhl's anomaly is right heart failure, which is associated with a high mortality rate. Recurrent sustained ventricular tachycardia has been rarely reported in this setting.[92] Conversely, ventricular tachyarrhythmias or sudden death are major components of ARVC. Adrenergic tone dependency of malignant arrhythmias characterizes ARVC and is uncommon in Uhl's anomaly. Although the pathologic features of Uhl's disease are unique, this entity remains affiliated with the right ventricular myocardial diseases.

Brugada Syndrome

ARVC should also be distinguished from the Brugada syndrome,[93,94] another clinical entity characterized by increased risk of syncope or cardiac arrest due to ventricular fibrillation, associated with right bundle branch block and ST-segment elevation in right precordial leads without any evidence of structural heart disease. However, the ST-segment elevation is inconsistently present and can be provoked pharmacologically with Class I antiarrhythmic drugs (ajmaline, procainamide, and flecainide). Occasionally, in patients diagnosed with the Brugada syndrome in whom routine diagnostic methods showed no abnormalities, MRI could suggest fatty replacement in the right ventricular infundibulum consistent with ARVC. Moreover, pathologic investigation in familial forms of Brugada syndrome reportedly disclosed adipose replacement of the right ventricular free wall.[95] Actually, mutations affecting the cardiac sodium channel gene (*SCN5A*) have been found in three small families and in individual patients. The gene is the same as that implicated in some forms of long QT syndrome (LQT3).[96] In the Brugada syndrome, the mutations identified apparently lead to a loss of function, whereas in LQT3, most cause a gain of function. Thus, LQT3 and the Brugada syndrome appear to be separate allelic disorders. Patients with the Brugada syndrome are mostly male and have a first arrhythmic event around their fourth decade. The recurrence rate of new arrhythmic events is as high as 40%. Pharmacologic treatment does not seem to protect effectively against relapses, and implantation of a cardioverter-defibrillator appears to be the only effective therapy to prevent sudden death. Finally, any relation of the Brugada syndrome to ARVC is currently conjectural.

Generalized Cardiomyopathy

Differentiation of ARVC from cardiomyopathy with predominant right ventricular dysfunction may be particularly difficult if the left ventricular ejection fraction is markedly reduced. In this situation attention may not be drawn to the right ventricular involvement as a primary cause of the disease. Unlike dilated cardiomyopathy, ARVC usually exhibits little or no progression of left ventricular systolic dysfunction.[7] Further evidence may be acquired by ECG and imaging techniques. In this view MRI is of peculiar interest because it provides insight into myocardial tissue composition. Ultimately, endomyocardial biopsy can be performed to search for the typical pathologic changes of ARVC. It is likely, however, that some biventricular forms of ARVC remain undetected. Their number among the cases of cardiomyopathy is unknown.

Natural History and Prognosis

Many problems exist regarding the natural history of ARVC. The true onset of the disease is unknown because a concealed phase probably precedes the symptomatic phase. Long-term follow-up studies are relatively few and selection bias may exist because most include patients with severe arrhythmias. The notion that the disease progresses tends to be accepted, but whether this process generally occurs or only affects subsets of patients is a matter of uncertainty. Ultimately, the left ventricle can be involved with subsequent biventricular failure. Actually, the factors underlying this evolution are unclear. Specific (perhaps genetic) characteristics may account for the particular course in the biventricular forms. Similarly, the progression toward heart failure is rarely seen and its bases are poorly understood.

Although the long-term prognosis for patients with ARVC appears to be more favorable than that for patients with ventricular tachyarrhythmias in the setting of ischemic heart disease or dilated cardiomyopathy, mortality rate due to sudden arrhythmic death and heart failure is significant.[39-42] Blomström-Lundqvist et al.[40] reported a 20% mortality rate after 8.8 years of follow-up in patients undergoing empiric antiarrhythmic treatment. Marcus et al.[5] reported a 17% mortality rate during long-term follow-up. Although patients with more concealed forms of the disease appear to carry a lower risk for serious arrhythmic event and cardiac arrest, sudden death has also been reported in this group of patients.[31]

Sudden arrhythmic death is an essential factor influencing the prognosis of the disease. Identification of risk factors is therefore a major step toward the prevention of sudden death. This issue remains controversial. Some studies failed to identify any predictor of sudden death in affected patients.[97] However, the lethal risk may be increased in patients with syncope and/or family history of sudden death. Bettini et al.[98] stressed the role of sustained or polymorphic ventricular arrhythmias and of left ventricular abnormalities. In a retrospective study on a cohort of 121 patients, Peters et al.[35] found that right ventricular dilatation and additional left ventricular abnormalities demonstrated by echocardiography and/or angiography, increased QRS duration ($\geq$110 ms), precordial T wave inversion beyond V_3, QT dispersion $\geq$50 ms, and JT dispersion $\geq$30 ms on the ECG were strong predictors of arrhythmic events.

In another report, Peters and Reil[63] were able to relate risk of sudden death to definite enlargement of the right ventricle, reduced global right ventricular ejection fraction (<40%), hypokinesia or akinesia of three or more right ventricular segments, end-diastolic/end-systolic out-pouchings in more than two segments, and inducible sustained ventricular arrhythmia during programmed ventricular stimulation. This subgroup of patients had a typical form of the disease with progressive worsening of right ventricular function and increasing electrical imbalance. However, strenuous exercise, and sport remained the most important precipitating factors.

Long-term follow-up data from clinical studies seem to indicate that ARVC is usually a progressive disease. The right ventricle may become more diffusely involved with time, leading to right-sided heart failure. Left ventricular impairment appears at all functional and morphologic stages of the disease, even in cases showing only slight or moderate right ventricular dysfunction. Heart failure tends to worsen progressively, and is more frequent with increasing age. In a series of patients reported by Pinamonti et al.,[45] presence of heart failure was found to be associated with increased mortality rate (50%) compared to patients with no symptoms or with arrhythmias (15%). In a series of patients with ARVC reported by Peters et al.,[30] heart failure (mostly right sided) appeared in 11% of patients over a follow-up period of 4 to 8 years.

In general, assessing prognosis in individual cases is almost impossible. Even severe pathologic forms with diffuse right ventricular involvement remain clinically stable over the long term. Right heart failure can be controlled for years with drug therapy. Conversely, survivors of cardiac arrest are likely to subsequently develop life-threatening events. The poor tolerance of the attacks in patients with episodes of sustained monomorphic ventricular tachycardia may be indicative of an unfavorable prognosis. Hemodynamic intolerance sometimes becomes manifest with time. Ventricular arrhythmias may then exhibit polymorphic patterns and faster rates. Despite the lack of definite evidence, an aggravating role of antiarrhythmic therapy is always possible. In fact, many patients suffer mostly from recurrent, moderately tolerated attacks that result in repeat hospitalizations. This contributes to a significantly reduced quality of life and also causes anxiety and psychological disorders. Most ARVC patients are young and hardly bear the impact of the disease on their daily life. Furthermore, the long-term administration of antiarrhythmic drugs and their inevitable side effects constitute an additional burden during the course of the disease.

Therapy

Although the outcome of right ventricular cardiomyopathy is often favorable, patients remain exposed during the long term to sudden arrhythmic death and the development of progressive heart failure. Thus, the notion of persisting risk must be kept in mind when selecting a therapeutic option. However, due to the rarity of the disease, the series reported in the literature are limited and the data that may provide bases for an appropriate management are insufficient. The clinical markers that predict outcome are under debate. Similarly, selection of therapy may have rational grounds, but commonly lacks scientific evidence. The treatment of patients with ARVC is basically empiric. Various strategies can ensue based on particular experiences. Like other aspects of the disease, therapy is a field of uncertainties, which leaves open the prospect for future studies. The following paragraphs are to be read as reflecting some consensus on the value and place of the available therapeutic options. This of course does not exclude the possibility of significant differences in the mode of management among centers.

Pharmacologic Therapy

Selection of a therapeutic strategy is dependent on the clinical presentation. An apparently benign presentation is that of a patient with frequent or complex ventricular ectopic activities combined with suggestive signs of right ventricular cardiomyopathy. This can occasionally be seen in the setting of familial forms of the disease. The subsequent arrhythmic risk is difficult to evaluate. The notion of underlying cardiomyopathy justifies further exploration of the significance of the clinical arrhythmia. Inducibility of sustained ventricular tachycardia following exercise stress testing or electrophysiologic study is supposedly related to the presence of a potentially malignant arrhythmogenic substrate. A positive response supports the use of prophylactic antiarrhythmic drug therapy despite the lack of definite evidence. In this view, an agent like sotalol, which combines Class III and β-blocking properties, might be preferred.[99] Class I antiarrhythmics can be rather envisaged in patients with bradycardia or intolerance to β-blockers. However, testing to initiate therapy may not be performed, since its value has not been established. Furthermore, whether the absence of inducible arrhythmias is associated with an event-free clinical course is far from certain. Due to these uncertainties, antiarrhythmic therapy can only be restricted to symptomatic forms. An alternative option consists of generalizing the prescription of drugs in order to counteract a well accepted but unpredictable risk. Thus, systematic β-blocking therapy has been recommended prophylactically,[100] although the benefit-risk ratio of this measure is unknown. In every case, sport activity must be proscribed.

Most frequently, the clinician deals with patients suffering from episodes of sustained ventricular tachyarrhythmia. Direct-current countershocks are the preferred method used to restore sinus rhythm. However, in patients with good cardiocirculatory status, administration of intravenous antiarrhythmics such as lidocaine, Class Ic, or Class III agents can be envisaged. The hemodynamic tolerance of the attacks is also used as a guide to select subsequent management. Following a first well-tolerated episode of tachycardia, drug therapy is licit. β-Blockers in particular should be considered, the arrhythmia being commonly dependent on increased adrenergic tone. Sotalol is the drug of choice due to its wide electrophysiologic spectrum. Besides blocking the β-adrenoreceptors, sotalol inhibits the outward potassium currents, which accounts for the lengthening of myocardial repolarization and refractoriness. In case of recurrent or poorly tolerated tachycardia, electrophysiologic testing is recommended to determine the appropriate antiarrhythmic agent, although the value of the guided approach in this setting is unproven. Suppression of ventricular arrhythmia inducibility is the endpoint. Class Ic antiarrhythmics and sotalol are more easily assessed than amiodarone using electrophysiologic techniques.[99] However, amiodarone, given empirically, remains a last resort option that may provide effective treatment of refractory arrhythmic recurrences.[92] Some investigators have also studied combination of antiarrhythmics.[99,100] Amiodarone may thus be associated with β-blockers or Class I agents, bearing in mind that any drug combination carries an increased risk of intolerance. Irrespective of the antiarrhythmic used, the long-term drug efficacy is unknown. However, the incidence of ventricular tachycardia recurrences appears to be low. In a prospective study on 81 patients with ARVC, Wichter et al.[99] evaluated the short- and long-term efficacy of antiarrhythmic drugs. In patients with inducible sustained ventricular tachycardia during programmed ventricular stimulation, sotalol suppressed the arrhythmia in 68% of patients, whereas Class Ia and Ib drugs were effective in only 6%, Class Ic drugs in 12%, and amiodarone in 15% of patients. Drug combination did not offer any additional benefit. In this group, nonfatal arrhythmia recurrence rate was 10% during a follow-up of 34 months. In patients with no electrically inducible ventricular arrhythmia, in whom Holter monitoring and exercise testing were used to assess drug action, sotalol was again most effective. Within 14 months, 12% of patients in this group had nonfatal arrhythmia recurrences. Moreover, the impact of drug therapy on sudden death risk is unclear. The parallel between drug control of sustained ventricular arrhythmias and prevention of sudden death remains to be established.

Radiofrequency Catheter Ablation

Radiofrequency catheter ablation has been proposed as an alternative therapy for patients with drug-refractory and hemodynamically stable sustained ventricular tachycardia.[101] As soon as resistance to drugs is apparent and impairs quality of life, catheter ablation must be considered. This technique has replaced direct-current ablation, which had been introduced for the treatment of ventricular tachycardia in 1983. Mapping and entrainment techniques (Figs. 14 and 15) can be used to characterize reentrant circuits and to guide ablation.[66,102] Acute suppression of tachycardia by current delivery at sites of diastolic activity is feasible. Isolation of critical areas by radiofrequency ablation has also been performed.[103] However, relevant series are limited and a definite knowledge of long-term results is lacking. Up to 50% recurrence rates have been reported during follow-up, with attacks of different morphology as compared to the initial arrhythmia. Ablation should be viewed as adjunctive treatment. Antiarrhythmic drug therapy is usually maintained. Potentiation of drug effect by ablation is possible. In patients in whom a cardioverter-defibrillator has been inserted, complementary catheter ablation may help to reduce the number of attacks and subsequent shocks. Moreover, potential hazards contraindicate ablation in those patients with severe right ventricular dysplasia. Marked thinning of the right ventricular muscle may then expose these patients to the risk of perforation. This should reinforce caution in using a therapeutic tool whose impact is still debated. The advent of antiarrhythmic devices has contributed to a further reduction in the role of ablation in the treatment of ARVC.

Surgical Disconnection of the Right Ventricle

Before catheter ablation, surgical procedures had been designed to treat drug-refractory patients with ARVC. The very first approach consisted of performing a single ventriculotomy at the site of earliest epicardial activation, as identified by intraoperative mapping, in order to interrupt local reentrant circuits.[4] However, new forms of ventricular tachycardia occurred frequently after surgery. Subsequently, total or partial disarticulation of the right ventricular free wall was described by Guiraudon et al.[104] and aimed at isolating the abnormal myocardial zones from the rest of the heart. The rationale for this method was twofold. First, by isolating the ventricles from each other, the procedure decreased the ventricular mass available for ventricular fibrillation. The other effect was to confine any ventricular tachycardia to the right ventricular free wall and to prevent the transmission of abnormal rhythms to the left ventricle. An adverse consequence was acute postoperative right ventricular failure that gradually resolved.[92] Results in terms of long-lasting suppression of ventricular tachycardia are poorly known. Furthermore, the progression of the disease is likely to counteract the early benefit of surgery. Thus, right ventricular disconnection has, for the most part, been abandoned. Again, the recent advances in device therapy have accelerated the decline of antiarrhythmic surgery.

Internal Cardioverter-Defibrillator

For patients with near-fatal arrhythmias and those who have survived cardiac arrest, the most effective safeguard against sudden cardiac death admittedly is the implantable cardioverter-defibrillator (ICD), even though there is no definitive evidence supporting this option. In the recurrent forms of sustained ventricular tachycardia, the availability of ICDs has radically changed the approach to refractory patients. In this case, the rationale of device therapy is based on the suppressibility of tachycardias by rapid pacing, shock delivery occurring as the last resort. The recourse to low-energy cardioversion as the first-intent approach is used with far less frequency, one reason being poor tolerance. In a series of 82 patients with ARVC reported by Breithardt et al.,[105] an ICD was implanted in 18 patients. Indications for ICD implantations consisted of drug-refractory malignant ventricular arrhythmias, previous cardiac arrest without inducible ventricular tachycardia or fibrillation, and failure of catheter ablation. During a follow-up of 17 months, 50% of patients received appropriate electrical therapy.

Although the perioperative complication rate is low, pacing thresholds may be higher and R wave amplitudes lower in patients with ARVC, thus requiring testing at two or more ventricular sites.[106] On the other hand, Link et al.[106] found no significant difference in defibrillation thresholds in ARVC patients compared to a cohort of control patients.

Thus, in addition to defibrillation, antitachycardia pacing can eliminate most tachycardias, thereby preventing life-threatening events and repeat hospitalizations. Moreover, combined drug therapy may be helpful for decreasing the frequency and rate of ventricular arrhythmia episodes. Additional recourse to catheter ablation is envisaged in case of too frequent, sustained arrhythmic episodes despite concomitant antiarrhythmics. Currently, the actual role of defibrillation therapy in ARVC is better defined. Expanding use of antitachyarrhythmia devices in ARVC has been facilitated by the advent of endocardial lead systems and also the lack of satisfactory alternatives in drug-refractory patients.

Treatment of ARVC Associated with Right or Biventricular Heart Failure

When heart failure is present because of severe right ventricular or biventricular systolic dysfunction, treatment is the same as for any patient with cardiac decompensation, and includes diuretics, angiotensin-converting enzyme inhibitors, digitalis, and, possibly, anticoagulant therapy. The occurrence of ventricular arrhythmia episodes may cause further aggravation, rendering the control of the disease increasingly complex. In this view, the deleterious role of antiarrhythmics must always be considered. Long-lasting stabilization is possible. However, patients with intractable heart failure are occasionally amenable to heart transplantation. Currently heart failure patients at high risk for sudden cardiac death, such as survivors from cardiac arrest or those with drug-refractory, malignant tachyarrhythmias, are not necessarily candidates for heart transplant if their hemodynamic status is well controlled; instead they have a cardioverter-defibrillator inserted.

Prevention

ARVC is a rare entity that is associated with a lethal risk. Any preventive approach to the disease is impaired by a number of problems. The clinical contours are imprecise, rendering the epidemiologic data questionable. The size of the pathologic population is unknown. Definite assessment of sudden death risk is accordingly impossible. However, among patients with known ARVC treated by drugs, the frequency of arrhythmic deaths can reportedly reach 2% to 3% per year. This provides a target for prevention measures. In the arrhythmologic literature, prevention applied to patients who have suffered from malignant arrhythmias or resuscitated cardiac arrest is improperly named "secondary." Currently, regarding the various antiarrhythmic options, any proof of their efficacy against sudden cardiac death risk is lacking. Implantable defibrillators may provide the most appropriate tool in this setting. Primary prevention concerns patients with the disease who have not yet experienced life-threatening events. Those patients who are at risk must be identified.

In fact, no indisputable markers could have been defined thus far. The notion of familial sudden death, recurrent syncope, or left ventricular involvement may be of significance. Furthermore, risk of sudden death due to ARVC is enhanced by intense sport activity. In this view, the subset of young competitive athletes is of peculiar interest. It is admitted that the disease in this context may actually be suspected on the basis of family history, arrhythmic prodromal symptoms, and electrocardiographic features. With effective screening including increased awareness of the disease, prevention of ARVC-related sudden death in young athletes appears to be a reasonable expectation. However, the field of prevention far exceeds that of competitive sport. The cost of any systematic prophylactic policy in the schools is likely to be exorbitant. Such an approach is impaired by the deficiencies of the tests associated with an unknown potential for erroneous responses. Assessment of risk in an individual who is suspected of ARVC on the basis of large-scale testing cannot rely on firm bases. Furthermore, the impact of prophylactic measures in this setting is conjectural. Finally, restricting the preventive approach to the relatives of patients who are treated for symptomatic ARVC seems to be more appropriate. Genetic tests should be added to the diagnostic evaluation. Again, the therapeutic implications for the suspected individuals have not been established. Sport cessation is a logical measure. Long-term β-blocking therapy may be advisable especially in a context of familial sudden death.

International Registry

Given the inherent uncertainties about the prevalence and the natural history of ARVC, as well as the limitations of current techniques to diagnose the disease or to evaluate the efficacy of therapeutic approaches, an international registry has been established by the Study Group on ARVD/C of the Working Group on Myocardial and Pericardial Diseases and Arrhythmias of the European Society of Cardiology and the Scientific Council on Cardiomyopathies of the World Health Federation, that officially started on January 1, 2001.[107] The objective of the ARVD/C International Registry is to follow up for more than 10 years a large patient population, with the following aims: to prospectively validate criteria for clinical diagnosis of ARVC, to assess the natural course of the disease in different clinical subgroups including asymptomatic family members, to identify groups at high risk for sudden death and poor prognosis, and to improve clinical management by evaluating long-term efficacy of empiric or test-guided antiarrhythmic agents or nonpharmacologic therapies. This project may also facilitate pathologic, molecular, and genetic research on the causes of the disease. Furthermore, availability of an international database should enhance awareness of this condition among cardiologists.

Conclusion

Despite remarkable advances in the understanding of ARVC in the last decades, much remains to be accomplished regarding the definition of the disease, the mechanisms underlying the pathophysiologic process, the clinical recognition with special reference to the diagnostic tests, the appraisal of prognosis, and the strategies of management. The pathologic characteristic of the disease is the myocardial infiltration by fatty tissue with or without fibrotic reaction. Replacement of ventricular muscle by fat affects exclusively, or predominantly, the right ventricular free wall. It is unclear whether fat results from programmed apoptosis or appears as a healing process following inflammatory phenomena. Disorganization of myocyte arrangement is assumedly responsible for fractionation of the excitation wave, slow conduction, and reentry. The notion of arrhythmogenicity belongs to the definition of the disease. Actually, occurrence of ventricular arrhythmias is commonly a starting point for identifying ARVC in the clinical setting, although latent forms do exist. The incidence and significance of asymptomatic ARVC are still unknown. This nosologic problem is further aggravated by the existence of biventricular forms that may erroneously suggest a dilated cardiomyopathy. Due to these uncertainties, consistent epidemiologic data are lacking. Thus, knowledge is mainly restricted to the arrhythmia patients. Even in this subset, definitive evidence for ARVC often cannot be obtained, particularly in cases of localized disease. No routine test is satisfactory and the new imaging tools under investigation must still prove their utility.

Even though in a significant number of patients the disease appears to be controlled by antiarrhythmic drug therapy, the clinical course carries a risk of sudden cardiac death. Sudden death may be the first manifestation of the disease in competitive athletes. Unfortunately, predictors of risk are missing. Sport is certainly a triggering factor. Drug-refractory, poorly tolerated sustained ventricular tachycardias may herald cardiac arrest. In the latter case, implantable defibrillation therapy has been invaluable. Device therapy has even become a privileged alternative in any recurrent form of ARVC. The management of the disease in asymptomatic patients remains a matter of debate. In familial forms, relatives of at-risk ARVC patients may be given β-blockers despite of the lack of definite evidence.

Genetics should open new doors for the identification and the care of patients with ARVC. Data are still sparse. Further progress is needed, as this field of investigation is only just emerging. A clarification of the genetic defects underlying the various phenotypes of the disease is expected. Furthermore, genetics is likely to shed new insight into pathogenesis of the disease. Therapeutic implications may ensue. Regardless, new exciting developments are awaited in the future.

References

1. Osler WLM. The Principles and Practice of Medicine. 6th ed. New York: D'Appleton; 1905:820.
2. Uhl HSM. A previously undescribed congenital malformation of the heart: almost total absence of the myocardium of the right ventricle: Bull Johns Hopkins Hospital. 1952;91:197-209.
3. Froment R, Perrin A, Loire R, et al. Ventricule droit papyracé du jeune adulte par dystrophie congénitale. A propos de 2 cas anatomo-cliniques et 3 cas cliniques. Arch Mal Coeur Vaiss 1968;61:477-503.
4. Fontaine G, Guiraudon G, Frank R, et al. Stimulation studies and epicardial mapping in ventricular tachycardia: study of mechanisms and selection for surgery. In: Kulbertus HE (ed): Reentrant Arrhythmias: Mechanisms and Treatment. Lancaster, PA: MTP Publishers; 1977:334-350.
5. Marcus FI, Fontaine G, Guiraudon G, et al. Right ventricular dysplasia: a report of 24 adult cases. Circulation 1982;65:384-399.
6. Thiene G, Nava A, Corrado D, et al. Right ventricular cardiomyopathy and sudden death in young people. N Engl J Med 1988;318:129-133.
7. Basso C, Thiene G, Corrado D, et al. Arrhythmogenic right ventricular cardiomyopathy: dysplasia, dystrophy, myocarditis? Circulation 1996;94:983-991.
8. Priori SG, Barhanin J, Hauer R, et al. Genetic and molecular basis of cardiac arrhythmias: impact on clinical management. Circulation 1999;99:518-528.
9. Loire R, Tabib A. Mort subite cardiaque inattendue. Bilan de 1000 autopsies. Arch Mal Coeur Vaiss 1996;1:13-18.
10. Burke AP, Farb A, Tashko G, Virmani R. Arrhythmogenic right ventricular cardiomyopathy and fatty replacement of the right ventricular myocardium: are they different diseases? Circulation 1998;97:1571-1580.

11. Mallat Z, Tedgui A, Fontaliran F, et al. Evidence of apoptosis in arrhythmogenic right ventricular dysplasia. N Engl J Med 1996;335:1190-1196.

12. Basso C, Thiene G, Nava A, Dalla Volta S. Arrhythmogenic right ventricular cardiomyopathy: a survey of the investigations at the University of Padua. Clin Cardiol 1997;20:333-336.

13. Fontaine G, Fontaliran F, Zerati O, et al. Fat in the heart. A feature unique to the human species? Observational reflection on an unsolved problem. Acta Cardiologica 1999;54:189-194.

14. Angelini A, Thiene G, Boffa G, et al. Endomyocardial biopsy in right ventricular cardiomyopathy. Int J Cardiol 1993;40:273-282.

15. Loire R, Tabib A. Arrhythmogenic right ventricular dysplasia and Uhl disease. Anatomic study of 100 cases after sudden death. Ann Pathol 1998;18:165-171.

16. Fontaine G, Guiraudon G, Frank R, et al. Dysplasie ventriculaire droite arythmogène et maladie de Uhl. Arch Mal Coeur 1982;4:361-372.

17. Richardson P, McKenna W, Bristow M, et al. Report of the 1995 World Health Organization/International Society and Federation of Cardiology Task Force on the Definition and Classification of Cardiomyopathies. Circulation 1996;93:841-842.

18. Rakover C, Rossi L, Fontaine G, et al. Familial arrhythmogenic right ventricular disease. Am J Cardiol 1986;58:377-378.

19. Nava A, Scognamiglio R, Thiene G, et al. A polymorphic form of familial arrhythmogenic right ventricular dysplasia. Am J Cardiol 1987;59:1405-1409.

20. Nava A, Thiene G, Canciani B, et al. Familial occurrence of right ventricular dysplasia: a study involving nine families. J Am Coll Cardiol 1988;12:1222-1228.

21. Fontaine G, Fontaliran F, Lascault G, et al. Dysplasie transmise et dysplasie acquise. Arch Mal Coeur 1990;83:915-920.

22. Thiene G, Corrado D, Nava A, et al. Right ventricular cardiomyopathy: is there evidence of an inflammatory etiology? Eur Heart J 1991;12(Suppl D):22-25.

23. Sabel KG, Blomström-Lundqvist C, Olsson SB, Enestrom S. Arrhythmogenic right ventricular dysplasia in brother and sister: is it related to myocarditis? Pediatr Cardiol 1990;11:113-116.

24. Hofmann R, Trappe HJ, Klein H, Kemmitz J. Chronic (or healed) myocarditis mimicking right ventricular dysplasia. Eur Heart J 1993;14:717-720.

25. Grumbach IM, Heim A, Vonhof S, et al. Coxakievirus genome in myocardium of patients with arrhythmogenic right ventricular dysplasia/cardiomyopathy. Cardiology 1998;89:241-245.

26. Matsumori A, Kawai C. Coxakievirus B3 perimyocarditis in BALB/c mice: experimental model of chronic perimyocarditis in the right ventricle. J Pathol 1980;131:97-106.

27. Basso C, Corrado D, Thiene G. Cardiovascular causes of sudden death in young individuals including athletes. Cardiol Rev 1999;3:127-135.

28. Sarubbi B, Ducceschi V, Santangelo L, Iacono A. Arrhythmias in patients with mechanical ventricular dysfunction and myocardial stretch: role of mechanoelectric feedback. Can J Cardiol 1998;14:245-252.

29. Wichter T, Hindricks G, Lerch H, et al. Regional myocardial dysinnervation in arrhythmogenic right ventricular cardiomyopathy: an analysis using ^{123}I-MIBG scintigraphy. Circulation 1994;89:667-683.

30. Peters S, Peters H, Thierfelder L. Heart failure in arrhythmogenic right ventricular dysplasia-cardiomyopathy. Int J Cardiol 1999;71:251-256.

31. Nava A, Thiene G, Canciani B, et al. Clinical profile of concealed form of arrhythmogenic right ventricular

cardiomyopathy with apparently idiopathic ventricular arrhythmias. Int J Cardiol 1992;35:195-206.

32. Leclercq JF, Potenza S, Maison-Blanche P, et al. Determinants of spontaneous occurrence of sustained monomorphic ventricular tachycardia in right ventricular dysplasia. J Am Coll Cardiol 1996;28:720-724.

33. Aouate P, Fontaliran F, Fontaine G, et al. Holter et mort subite. Intérêt dans un cas de dysplasie ventriculaire droite arrythmogène. Arch Mal Coeur Vaiss 1993;86:363-367.

34. Kullo IJ, Edwards WD, Seward JB. Right ventricular dysplasia: the Mayo Clinic experience. Mayo Clin Proc 1995;70:541-548.

35. Peters S, Peters H, Thierfelder L. Risk stratification of sudden cardiac death and malignant ventricular arrhythmias in right ventricular dysplasia-cardiomyopathy. Int J Cardiol 1999;71:243-250.

36. Corrado D, Basso C, Thiene G. Sudden cardiac death in young people with apparently normal heart. Cardiovasc Res 2000;50:399-408.

37. Burke AP, Farb A, Virmani R, et al. Sports-related and non sports-related sudden cardiac death in young adults. Am Heart J 1991;121:568-575.

38. Maron BJ, Shirani J, Poliac LC, et al. Sudden death in young competitive athletes: clinical, demographic and pathological profile. JAMA 1996;276:199-204.

39. Reiter MJ, Warren M, Smith PD, et al. Clinical spectrum of ventricular tachycardia with left bundle branch block morphology. Am J Cardiol 1983;51:113-121.

40. Blomström-Lundqvist C, Sabel KG, Olsson SB. A long-term follow-up of 15 patients with arrhythmogenic

right ventricular dysplasia. Br Heart J 1987;58:477-488.

41. Leclercq JF, Coumel P. Characteristics, prognosis and treatment of the ventricular arrhythmias of right ventricular dysplasia. Eur Heart J 1989;10(Suppl D):61-77.

42. Canu G, Atallah G, Claudel JP, et al. Pronostic et évolution à long terme de la dysplasie arrythmogène du ventricule droit. Arch Mal Coeur Vaiss 1993;86:41-48.

43. Tonet J, Castro Miranda R, Iwa T, et al. Frequency of supraventricular tachyarrhythmias in arrhythmogenic right ventricular dysplasia. Am J Cardiol 1991;67:1153.

44. Akazawa H, Ikeda U, Minezaki K, et al. Right ventricular dysplasia with complete atrioventricular block: necessity and limitation of left ventricular epicardial pacing. Clin Cardiol 1998;21:604-606.

45. Pinamonti B, Lenarda A, Sinagra G, et al. Long-term evolution of right ventricular dysplasia-cardiomyopathy. Am Heart J 1995;129:412-415.

46. Fontaine G, Frank R, Guiraudon G, et al. Signification des troubles de conduction intraventriculaires observés dans la dysplasie ventriculaire droite arythmogène. Arch Mal Coeur 1984;77:872-879.

47. Nemec J, Edwards BS, Osborn, MJ, Edwards WD. Arrhythmogenic right ventricular dysplasia masquerading as dilated cardiomyopathy. Am J Cardiol 1999;84:237-239.

48. Pinamonti B, Sinagra G, Salvi A, et al. Left ventricular involvement in right ventricular dysplasia. Am Heart J 1992;123:711-724.

49. Guttierez PS, Ferreira SMF, Lopes EA, et al. Intramural coronary vessels in partial absence of the myocar-

dium of the right ventricle. Am J Cardiol 1989;63:1152-1154.

50. Fontaine G, Umemura J, Di Donna P, et al. La durée des complexes QRS dans la dysplasie ventriculaire droite arythmogène. Un nouveau marqueur diagnostic non invasif. Ann Cardiol Angeiol 1993;42:399-405.

51. Metzger JT, de Chillou C, Cheiex E, et al. Value of the 12-lead electrocardiogram in arrhythmogenic right ventricular dysplasia, and absence of correlation with echocardiographic findings. Am J Cardiol 1993;72: 964-967.

52. Fontaine G, Piot O, Sohal P, et al. Dérivations en précordiales droites et mort subite. Relation avec la dysplasie ventriculaire droite arythmogène. Arch Mal Coeur 1996;89:1323-1328.

53. Benn M, Hansen PS, Pedersen AK. QT dispersion in patients with arrhythmogenic right ventricular dysplasia. Eur Heart J 1999;20:764-770.

54. Jaoude SA, Leclercq JF, Coumel P. Progressive ECG changes in arrhythmogenic right ventricular disease. Eur Heart J 1996;17:1717-1722.

55. Marcus FI, Fontaine G. Arrhythmogenic right ventricular dysplasia/cardiomyopathy: a review. Pacing Clin Electrophysiol 1995;18:1298-1314.

56. Toyofuku M, Takaki H, Sunagawa K, et al. Exercise-induced ST elevation in patients with arrhythmogenic right ventricular dysplasia. J Electrocardiol 1999;32:1-5.

57. Mehta D, Goldman M, David O, Gomes JA. Value of quantitative measurement of signal-averaged electrocardiographic variable in arrhythmogenic right ventricular dysplasia: correlation with echocardio-

graphic right ventricular cavity dimensions. J Am Coll Cardiol 1996;28:713-719.

58. Nava A, Folino F, Bauce B, et al. Signal-averaged electrocardiogram in patients with arrhythmogenic right ventricular cardiomyopathy and ventricular arrhythmias. Eur Heart J 2000;21:58-65.

59. Turini P, Angelini A, Thiene G, et al. Late potentials and ventricular arrhythmias in arrhythmogenic right ventricular cardiomyopathy. Am J Cardiol 1999;83: 1214-1219.

60. Hermida JS, Minassian A, Jarry G, et al. Familial incidence of late ventricular potentials and electrocardiographic abnormalities in arrhythmogenic right ventricular dysplasia. Am J Cardiol 1997;79:1375-1380.

61. Haïssaguerre M, Le Metayer P, D'Ivernois C, et al. Distinctive response of arrhythmogenic right ventricular disease to high dose isoproterenol. Pacing Clin Electrophysiol 1990;13(Pt. II):2119-2126.

62. DiBiase M, Favale V, Massari G, et al. Programmed stimulation in patients with minor forms of right ventricular dysplasia. Eur Heart J 1989;10(Suppl D):49-53.

63. Peters S, Reil H. Risk factors of cardiac arrest in arrhythmogenic right ventricular dysplasia. Eur Heart J 1995;16:77-80.

64. Panidis IP, Greenspan AM, Mintz GS, Ross J Jr. Inducible ventricular fibrillation in arrhythmogenic right ventricular dysplasia. Am Heart J 1985;110:1067-1069.

65. Rosenfeld LE, Batsford WP. Intraventricular Wenckebach conduction and localized reentry in a case of right ventricular dysplasia with recurrent ventricular tachycardia. J Am Coll Cardiol 1983;2:585-591.

66. Ellison KE, Friedman PL, Ganz LI, Stevenson WG. Entrainment mapping and radiofrequency ablation of ventricular tachycardia in right ventricular dysplasia. J Am Coll Cardiol 1998;32:724-728.

67. Brembilla-Perrot B, Jacquemein L, Houplon P, et al. Increased atrial vulnerability in arrhythmogenic right ventricular disease. Am Heart J 1998;135:748-754.

68. Scognamiglio R, Fasoli G, Nava A, et al. Contribution of cross-sectional echocardiography to the diagnosis of right ventricular dysplasia at the asymptomatic stage. Eur Heart J 1989;10:538-542.

69. Fontaine G, Fontaliran F, Hébert JL, et al. Arrhythmogenic right ventricular dysplasia. Ann Rev Med 1999;50:17-35.

70. Foale RA, Nihoyannopoulos P, McKenna WJ, et al. Echocardiographic measurement of the normal adult right ventricle. Br Heart J 1986;56:33-44.

71. Fontaine G, Fontaliran F, Frank R. Arrhythmogenic right ventricular cardiomyopathies. Clinical forms and main differential diagnoses (editorial). Circulation 1998;97:1532-1535.

72. De Piccoli B, Rigo F, Caprioglio F, et al. The usefulness of transesophageal echocardiography in the diagnosis of arrhythmogenic right ventricular cardiomyopathy. G Ital Cardiol 1993;23:247-259.

73. Angelini A, Basso C, Nava A, Thiene G. Endomyocardial biopsy in arrhythmogenic right ventricular cardiomyopathy. Am Heart J 1996;132:203-206.

74. Dobrinski G, Werdiere C, Fontaine G, et al. Diagnostic angiographique des dysplasies ventriculaires droites. Arch Mal Coeur 1985;78:544-551.

75. Blomström-Lundqvist C, Selin K, Jonsson R, et al. Cardioangiographic findings in patients with arrhyth-

mogenic right ventricular dysplasia. Br Heart J 1988;59:556-563.

76. Daliento L, Rizzoli G, Thiene G, et al. Diagnostic accuracy of right ventriculography in arrhythmogenic right ventricular cardiomyopathy. Am J Cardiol 1990;66:741-745.

77. Pavel D, Byrom E, Law W, et al. Detection and quantification of regional wall motion abnormalities using phase analysis of equilibrium gated cardiac studies. Clin Nucl Med 1983;8:315-321.

78. Bourguignon MH, Sebag C, Le Guludec D, et al. Arrhythmogenic right ventricular dysplasia demonstrated by phase mapping of gated equilibrium radioventriculography. Am Heart J 1986;111:997-1000.

79. Le Guludec D, Slama MS, Frank R, et al. Evaluation of radionuclide angiography in diagnosis of arrhythmogenic right ventricular cardiomyopathy. J Am Coll Cardiol 1995;26:1476-1483.

80. Casset-Senon D, Philippe L, Babuty D, et al. Diagnosis of arrhythmogenic right ventricular cardiomyopathy by Fourier analysis of gated blood pool single-photon emission tomography. Am J Cardiol 1998;82:1399-1404.

81. Daou D, Lebtahi R, Faraggi M, et al. Cardiac gated equilibrium radionuclide angiography and multiharmonic Fourier phase analysis: optimal acquisition parameters in right ventricular cardiomyopathy. J Nucl Cardiol 1999;6:429-437.

82. Markiewicz W, Sechtem U, Higgins CB. Evaluation of the right ventricle by magnetic resonance imaging. Am Heart J 1987;113:8-15.

83. Molinari F, Sardanelli F, Gaita F, et al. Right ventricular dysplasia as a generalized cardiomyopathy? Find-

ings on magnetic resonance imaging. Eur Heart J 1995;16:1619-1624.

84. Gill JS, Rowland E, De Belder M, et al. Cardiac abnormalities not visualized by echocardiography and angiography are detected by magnetic resonance imaging in patients with idiopathic ventricular tachycardia (abstract). Eur Heart J 1993;14:7A.

85. Rampazzo A, Nava A, Danieli GA, et al. The gene for arrhythmogenic right ventricular cardiomyopathy maps to chromosome 14q23-q24. Hum Mol Genet 1994;3:959-962.

86. Rampazzo A, Nava A, Erne P, et al. A new locus for arrhythmogenic right ventricular cardiomyopathy maps to chromosome 1q42-q43. Hum Mol Genet 1995;4:2151-2154.

87. Rampazzo A, Nava A, Miorin M, et al. A new locus for arrhythmogenic right ventricular cardiomyopathy (ARVD4) maps to chromosome 2q32. Genomics 1997;45:259-263.

88. Ahmad F, Li D, Karibe A, et al. Localization of a gene responsible for arrhythmogenic right ventricular dysplasia to chromosome 3p23. Circulation 1998;98:2791-2795.

89. Coonar AS, Protonotarius N, Tsatsopoulou A, et al. Gene for arrhythmogenic right ventricular cardiomyopathy with diffuse nonepidermolytic palmoplantar keratoderma and woolly hair (Naxos disease) maps to chromosome 17q21. Circulation 1998;97:2049-2058.

90. McKenna WJ, Thiene G, Nava A, et al. Diagnosis of arrhythmogenic right ventricular dysplasia/cardiomyopathy. Br Heart J 1994;71:215-218.

91. Carlson MD, White RD, Throhman RG, et al. Right ventricular outflow tract ventricular tachycardia: de-

tection of previously unrecognised anatomic abnormalities using cine magnetic resonance imaging. J Am Coll Cardiol 1994;24:720-727.

92. Marcus FI, Fontaine G. Arrhythmogenic right ventricular dysplasia/cardiomyopathy: a review. Pacing Clin Electrophysiol 1995;18:1298-1314.

93. Brugada J, Brugada P. Right bundle branch block, persistent ST segment elevation and sudden cardiac death: a distinct clinical and electrocardiographic syndrome—A multicenter report. J Am Coll Cardiol 1992;20:1391-1396.

94. Alings M, Wilde A. "Brugada" syndrome. Clinical data and suggested pathophysiological mechanism. Circulation 1999;99:666-673.

95. Corrado D, Nava A, Buja G, et al. Familial cardiomyopathy underlies syndrome of right bundle branch block. ST segment elevation and sudden death. J Am Coll Cardiol 1996;27:443-448.

96. Chen Q, Kirsch GE, Zhang D, et al. Genetic basis and molecular mechanism for idiopathic ventricular fibrillation. Nature 1998;392:293-294.

97. Leclercq JF, Denjoy I, Maison-Blanche P, et al. Valeur de l'electrocardiographie haute amplification chez les sujets ayant des troubles du rhythme ventriculaire sur coeur apparemment sain. Arch Mal Coeur Vaiss 1992;85:831-837.

98. Bettini R, Furlanello F, Vergara G, et al. Arrhythmologic study of 50 patients with arrhythmogenic disease of the right ventricle: prognostic implications. G Ital Cardiol 1989;19:567-579.

99. Wichter T, Borggrefe M, Haverkamp W, et al. Efficacy of antiarrhythmic drugs in patients with arrhythmogenic right ventricular disease. Results in patients

with inducible and noninducible ventricular tachycardia. Circulation 1992;86:29-37.

100. Fontaine G, Zenati O, Tonet J, et al. The treatment of ventricular arrhythmias. In: Nava A, Rossi L, Thiene G (eds): Arrhythmogenic Right Ventricular Cardiomyopathy-Dysplasia. Amsterdam: Elsevier; 1997:315.

101. Feld GK. Expanding indications for radiofrequency catheter ablation: ventricular tachycardia in association with right ventricular dysplasia. J Am Coll Cardiol 1998;32:729-731.

102. Harada T, Aonuma K, Yamauchi Y, et al. Catheter ablation of ventricular tachycardia in patients with right ventricular dysplasia: identification of target sites by entrainment mapping techniques. Pacing Clin Electrophysiol 1998;21(Pt. II):2547-2550.

103. Fukushima K, Emori T, Morita H, et al. Ablation of ventricular tachycardia by isolating the critical site in a patient with arrhythmogenic right ventricular cardiomyopathy. J Cardiovasc Electrophysiol 2000;11:102-105.

104. Guiraudon GM, Klein GJ, Gulamhusein S, et al. Total disconnection of the right ventricular free wall: surgical treatment of right ventricular tachycardia associated with right ventricular dysplasia. Circulation 1983;67:463-470.

105. Breithardt G, Wichter T, Haverkamp W, et al. Implantable cardioverter defibrillator therapy in patients with arrhythmogenic right ventricular cardiomyopathy, long QT syndrome or no structural heart disease. Am Heart J 1994;127:1151-1158.

106. Link MS, Wang PJ, Haugh CJ, et al. Arrhythmogenic right ventricular dysplasia: clinical results with im-

plantable cardioverter defibrillators. J Interv Card Electrophysiol 1997;1:41-48.

107. Corrado D, Fontaine G, Marcus FI, et al. Arrhythmogenic right ventricular dysplasia/cardiomyopathy: need for an international registry. Circulation 2000;101:1-6.

Index

Arrhythmogenic right ventricular cardiomyopathy (ARVC)
arrhythmogenic substrate of, 3
clinical picture of, 3
coexisting left ventricle damage, 3
definition of, 2–4
fatty histologic form of, 9, 11, 73–74
fatty infiltration of right ventricle of normal hearts, 11–12
fibrofatty histologic form, 7–9, 10, 73–74
limits of pathologic diagnosis, 11–12
myocarditis associated with fibrofatty histologic form, 8, 9
right ventricular anomaly of, 2
"Arrhythmogenic right ventricular dysplasia" (ARVD), 2

Becker's disease, 13

Clinical approach to ARVC, 55–57, 58
Clinical presentation of ARVC
associated with sudden cardiac death, 14, 22, 74
atrial arrhythmias in, 23–24
atrioventricular conduction in, 24
chest pain in, 26–27
Coxsackie virus in ARVC myocardium, 14
fatigue, palpitations, and/or syncope in, 16, 22, 23, 24, 26, 62
with heart failure, 16, 24, 26, 63
latent forms in, 27
misdiagnosis of "idiopathic ventricular arrhythmias," 16
occurrence with emotion or exercise, 15, 22, 63, 66, 74
role of drug-induced proarrhythmias, 23, 74

89

sick sinus syndrome in, 24, 25
sudden cardiac death due to ventricular fibrillation, 22–23
variable range of symptoms and modes of expression, 14, 74
ventricular ectopies/ tachycardia in, 16–22
ventricular rhythm disorders associated with, 15–23

Diagnostic criteria for ARVC, 56–57, 58
Diagnostic tools
chest X-ray, 28, 29
ECG in sinus rhythm, 17, 18, 25, 28–33, 56, 61
echocardiographic findings, 43–45, 55
electrophysiologic study, 39–43, 65
endomyocardial biopsy, 46, 55
exercise stress test, 33–35, 56, 65
gated blood-pool single-photon emission tomography (GBP-SPECT), 50, 51, 52
genetics studies and family history, 53–55, 62, 75

I-meta-iodobenzylguanidine (I-MIBG) scintigraphy, 50, 53
isoproterenol testing, 38–39, 41, 56
magnetic resonance imaging (MRI), 53, 54, 56, 61
physical examination, 27–28
radionuclide angiography and computed tomography, 47, 49–53, 56
right contrast ventriculography, 46–47, 48
signal-averaged ECG, 35–38, 56
Differential diagnosis
Brugada syndrome, 59–60
cardiac sodium channel gene (SCN5A), 60
generalized cardiomyopathy, 60–61
right ventricular outflow tract tachycardia, 57, 59
Uhl's disease, 59
Duchenne's disease, 13

Epidemiology of ARVC, 4–5
ARVC-related sudden cardiac death, 4
incidence and prevalence of ARVC, 4

European Society of Cardiology, 56, 73

Genetics and positive family history in ARVC cases, 53–55, 62, 75

Heart failure, ARVC associated with, 5, 16, 24, 26, 63

International registry for ARVC
  ARVD/C International Registry, 73
  European Society of Cardiology, 73
  Scientific Council on Cardiomyopathies, 73
  Study Group on ARVD/C, 73
  Working Group on Myocardial and Pericardial Diseases, 73
  World Health Federation, 73
International Society and Federation of Cardiology, 56

Natural history and prognosis
  concealed onset of ARVC, 61
  long-term follow-up data, 63

mortality rate from sudden cardiac death, 62

"Parchment heart," 1
Pathogenesis of ARVC
  degenerative theory in, 13
  as healing process following myocarditis, 13
  role of inflammation theory, 13
  Uhl's description of anomaly, 12
Pathology of ARVC
  cardiac muscle replaced by fat and fibrosis, 6–11
  histopathology, 6–11
  macroscopic aspect, 5–6
  "triangle of dysplasia," 5
Prevention of arrhythmogenic right ventricular cardiomyopathy (ARVC), 71–72

Scientific Council of Cardiomyopathies, 56, 73
Sudden cardiac death, ARVC-related, 4, 14, 22, 62, 74

Therapy for ARVC
  implantable cardioverter-defibrillator (ICD), 69–70, 74

pharmacologic therapy,
65–67
radiofrequency catheter
ablation, 67–68
surgical disconnection
of right ventricle, 68–
69
treatment associated
with right or biventri-
cular heart failure,
70–71

Working Group on Myocar-
dial and Pericardial Dis-
eases, 56, 73